# CLINICAL NEUROLOGY
# MADE EASY®

# CLINICAL NEUROLOGY MADE EASY®

**HV Srinivas**
MD (Gen) MD (Neurology)
Consultant Neurologist
Agadi Hospital and Sagar Hospital, Bengaluru
Former Visiting Consultant and Postgraduate Teacher for
DNB (Neurology)
Department of Neurology
Narayana Institute of Neurosciences
Bengaluru, Karnataka, India

*Forewords*
**BS Singhal**
**M Maiya**

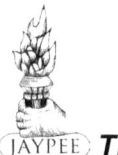

JAYPEE **The Health Sciences Publisher**
New Delhi | London | Panama

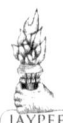 **Jaypee Brothers Medical Publishers (P) Ltd.**

**Headquarters**
Jaypee Brothers Medical Publishers (P) Ltd.
4838/24, Ansari Road, Daryaganj
New Delhi 110 002, India
Phone: +91-11-43574357
Fax: +91-11-43574314
E-mail: jaypee@jaypeebrothers.com

**Overseas Offices**

JP Medical Ltd.
83 Victoria Street, London
SW1H 0HW (UK)
Phone: +44-20 3170 8910
Fax: +44(0)20 3008 6180
E-mail: info@jpmedpub.com

Jaypee-Highlights Medical Publishers Inc.
City of Knowledge, Bld. 235, 2nd Floor, Clayton
Panama City, Panama
Phone: +1 507-301-0496
Fax: +1 507-301-0499
E-mail: cservice@jphmedical.com

Jaypee Brothers Medical Publishers (P) Ltd.
17/1-B, Babar Road, Block-B, Shyamoli
Mohammadpur, Dhaka-1207
Bangladesh
Mobile: +08801912003485
E-mail: jaypeedhaka@gmail.com

Jaypee Brothers Medical Publishers (P) Ltd.
Bhotahity, Kathmandu, Nepal
Phone: +977-9741283608
E-mail: kathmandu@jaypeebrothers.com

Website: www.jaypeebrothers.com
Website: www.jaypeedigital.com

© 2018, Jaypee Brothers Medical Publishers

The views and opinions expressed in this book are solely those of the original contributor(s)/author(s) and do not necessarily represent those of editor(s) of the book.

All rights reserved. No part of this publication may be reproduced, stored or transmitted in any form or by any means, electronic, mechanical, photocopying, recording or otherwise, without the prior permission in writing of the publishers.

All brand names and product names used in this book are trade names, service marks, trademarks or registered trademarks of their respective owners. The publisher is not associated with any product or vendor mentioned in this book.

Medical knowledge and practice change constantly. This book is designed to provide accurate, authoritative information about the subject matter in question. However, readers are advised to check the most current information available on procedures included and check information from the manufacturer of each product to be administered, to verify the recommended dose, formula, method and duration of administration, adverse effects and contraindications. It is the responsibility of the practitioner to take all appropriate safety precautions. Neither the publisher nor the author(s)/editor(s) assume any liability for any injury and/or damage to persons or property arising from or related to use of material in this book.

This book is sold on the understanding that the publisher is not engaged in providing professional medical services. If such advice or services are required, the services of a competent medical professional should be sought.

Every effort has been made where necessary to contact holders of copyright to obtain permission to reproduce copyright material. If any have been inadvertently overlooked, the publisher will be pleased to make the necessary arrangements at the first opportunity. The **CD/DVD-ROM** (if any) provided in the sealed envelope with this book is complimentary and free of cost. **Not meant for sale.**

**Inquiries for bulk sales may be solicited at**: jaypee@jaypeebrothers.com

*Clinical Neurology Made Easy®*

*First Edition:* **2018**

**ISBN:** 978-93-5270-251-0

Printed at

### Dedicated to

*My students for their abiding interest to learn*
*My wife Dr Pushpa Srinivas for her unstinted cooperation to complete this book*
*My family—my son Sachin, daughter Minoti and son-in-law Mukund*
*My sweet little granddaughters Esha, Mihika and Minal*

# Foreword

I am indeed honored to write the foreword for the book *Clinical Neurology Made Easy*. Today the technological advances in Neurology have made an immense contribution to the understanding of neurological diseases and helped in arriving at the diagnosis. Nevertheless they cannot and should not take us away from the basic clinical approach which gives due importance to the history (which also increases level of communication and empathy with the patient) and clinical findings to lead us to appropriate investigations for the diagnosis. More importantly, many investigations have incidental findings which may not have any clinical significance, e.g. in cervical disc prolapse, lumbar disc prolapse and lacunar infarcts. One starts treating the images rather than the patient!

This book emphasizes once again that clinical neurology is the bottom line for proper diagnosis. It is a reminder that all investigations should be a servant to the physician and not the master! Common neurological disorders like headache, giddiness and tremors, seen not only by neurologists but also by primary care physicians, family physicians and specialists are well covered in this book. The symptom-wise approach with relevant tables and case illustrations will be very helpful to the reader. Generally in a book 'when to do' a particular investigation will be mentioned, but in this book the author also emphasizes on 'when not to do' a particular investigation. The book is a ready-reckoner for step-wise diagnostic approach and management of common conditions. The escalating health cost should bring attention to the need for minimum necessary investigations and minimum cost effective prescriptions.

I have enjoyed reading the book by Dr HV Srinivas, well known for his impeccable clinical acumen. It is a welcome addition to academic neurology with its emphasis on a sound clinical approach and I would highly recommend it to all neurologists and physicians.

**Dr BS Singhal** MD FRCP
Director of Neurology
Bombay Hospital Institute of Medical Sciences
Mumbai, Maharashtra, India

# Foreword

It is a privilege and honor to write the foreword for *Clinical Neurology Made Easy* authored by Dr HV Srinivas.

The science of medicine is progressing at an unprecedented rate along with high technology for the last few decades. A third of what we know today becomes obsolete after 10 to 15 years. The advancement in the knowledge of the diseases affecting the various systems in the body is responsible for establishment of 'Super Speciality' (? Subspeciality) departments/clinics like Neurology, Cardiology, Nephrology, Pulmonology, etc. managed by superspecialists.

However, the majority of the problems in medicine is managed by General Practitioners and Internists because of their easy accessibility. Yet one observes certain amount of inertia and hesitation on the part of General Practitioners and Internists to accept and manage the patients with common neurological disorders. It may be due to inadequate training in basic clinical approach, lack of confidence, unsatisfactory results of several conditions and costly investigations. Hence, the book on *Clinical Neurology Made Easy* written by Dr HV Srinivas, an experienced teacher who has been teaching postgraduate students in Medicine for more than 35 years, voluntarily, is a welcome addition to the armamentarium of clinicians.

The book contains common neurological conditions which can be managed by primary care physicians and internists. Only a few cases need a reference to a neurologist. The common diseases described here are Cerebrovascular Stroke, Parkinson's Disease, Epilepsy, Back and Neck Pain, Gait Imbalances, etc. with illustrative cases and tables for quick reference. Even symptom-oriented diseases like Tension Headache, Migraine, Giddiness and Dementia are also dealt with.

The book emphasizes the supremacy of clinical neurology and bedside examination in the era of high-tech medicine. Listening to the history of patient indicates the diagnosis more often than costly investigations. History taking also reveals the personality and attitude of the patient which is essential for the management of the disease. It is Sir William Osler who said 'It is more important to know what patient has the disease than what disease the patient has'.

Undoubtedly the book achieves its objective of *Clinical Neurology Made Easy* and Dr HV Srinivas is eminently suited for this as an author. The book is a welcome addition to be used as a 'ready reckoner' while practicing medicine.

**Dr M Maiya**
MBBS FRCP (Lond) FRCP (Edin)
FRCP (GLASG), FICC (Ind) FICP (Ind)
Consultant Physician and
Former Professor of Medicine
Bengaluru, Karnataka, India

# Preface

A large number of common neurological disorders are seen by primary care physicians and internists. In fact, there is no need for a neurologist to see all such cases. Methodical evaluation is the key to proper diagnosis and management. Evaluation is by clinical method and investigations are asked for *only when necessary*. With technological advances, life has become easier but the brain is being rested and rusted! In fact, there is a need to remind people that the brain is also an app—start using it! The advances in technology are making inroads into medical field with the result that clinical medicine is slowly dying.

It is generally perceived that an MR scan will result in an accurate diagnosis. However, when the MR scan is normal and patient is not normal, the patient is referred to a neurologist, resulting in a new category of 'MR negative neurologists'. Of course, if the MR scan shows some abnormality, as reported by the radiologist, it is promptly treated forgetting that it may not be causative but purely incidental. The point highlighted here is that some of the common neurological disorders like tension headache, migraine, epilepsy, Parkinson's disease and dementia are entirely based on the clinical diagnosis and there are *no investigations to confirm the diagnosis*.

This book is an attempt to emphasize in no uncertain terms that clinical neurology is supreme, more so in this era of technological advances. If the MR findings are at variance with the clinical diagnosis, the clinical diagnosis should be reviewed so as to confirm it. The old advice 'listen to the patient, he is telling the diagnosis' is very true, even today. Due to lack of time there is no proper history taking and in order to save time, investigations are quickly ordered to get a diagnosis. Technology and investigation must remain a servant of the clinician—not the master.

This book deals with symptom-related topics like headache, giddiness and contains tables for quick reference. Hopefully, this book will be a ready-reckoner in the busy OPD practice. Illustrated case histories with step-wise diagnosis are provided to help the clinician think and analyze the symptoms accurately.

Though I have been in private practice, my passion for teaching prompted me to take weekly classes for postgraduate students in medicine for more than 35 years—a record by any standard. The voluntary participation of the students in large numbers in these classes has given me a lot of satisfaction and encouragement.

This book is a culmination of my clinical teaching realizing the lacunae, fear, myths and misunderstanding of the subject. In our country neurology training is grossly inadequate—at best perfunctory to internists. This book is a guide for approach to diagnosis, appropriate investigations and proper management of common neurological problems. Clinical discussions and differential diagnosis in this book are not all inclusive but only cover the common disorders. For further information the reader can refer to standard books.

'Common conditions are common' is true, as much for students, as for professors of Neurology, and is also the basis of good clinical practice. Once the common diseases are ruled out, one can refer to books for the not- so-common disorders.

Every clinician's aim is to look for a treatable condition—however atypical the presentation may be. I have emphasized on the treatable conditions and have not touched upon several exotic conditions/diagnosis which even if missed do not really matter for the patients' prognosis or management. For example, one should not miss the treatable polymyositis but it does not matter if a type of muscular dystrophy is missed. Similarly, a treatable dementia due to vitamin B12 deficiency or thyroid disorder; myopathy due to vitamin D deficiency should not be missed.

Healthcare is now a profitable industry resulting in unnecessary and over investigations adding to the cost and misery of patients. So, the practice of prescribing drugs of dubious value and expensive branded drugs, in place of cost effective generic drugs. Emphasis is placed on minimum and required investigations and useful and necessary medication.

I have made an attempt to make clinical neurology easy—easy to understand and practice. Hope it meets the expectations.

**HV Srinivas**

# Acknowledgments

The idea of writing this book is a by-product of my continued interaction with postgraduate students in medicine and primary care physicians during the last 36 years. I have understood the lacunae of postgraduate students when faced with common neurological disorders, due to lack of adequate neurology training during the postgraduate course. This book is a guide to help out students and consultants in general medicine to approach neurological problems in a methodical way.

But for the interest of the student population, there would not have been any idea of writing this book!

My sincere thanks to Dr BS Singhal and Dr M Maiya for writing the foreword.

My sincere thanks to Mr Sreeram Rama Chandran (Architect, Designer and Artist), who has drawn a number of sketches which have been incorporated in this book.

I thank Ms Meena Chandramohan for copyediting the book.

I thank Dr Anand and Ms Vinutha of Medall Clumax Diagnostic Centre, Jayanagar for the images incorporated here.

Finally, I acknowledge the sincere hard work put up by my secretary Ms Theresa Pinto for typing several drafts ungrudgingly before it took the final shape.

# Contents

| | |
|---|---|
| Foreword 1 | vii |
| Foreword 2 | ix |
| Preface | xi |
| Acknowledgments | xiii |
| 1. Introduction | 1 |
| 2. History | 6 |
| 3. Neurological Examination | 11 |
| 4. Investigations | 19 |
| 5. Headache | 31 |
| 6. Dizziness/Vertigo | 41 |
| 7. Neck Pain | 48 |
| 8. Back Pain | 55 |
| 9. Blurring of Vision, Double Vision | 60 |
| 10. Syncope/Drop Attacks | 69 |
| 11. Seizure/Epilepsy | 73 |
| 12. Difficulty to Talk | 83 |
| 13. Difficulty to Write | 86 |
| 14. Gait Imbalance | 87 |
| 15. Motor Weakness and Paraplegia | 95 |
| 16. Neurogenic Bladder | 112 |
| 17. Difficulty to get up from Squatting/Climbing Stairs | 118 |
| 18. Pins/Needles in Feet | 129 |
| 19. Tremors | 137 |
| 20. Parkinson's Disease | 140 |
| 21. Memory Impairment/Dementia | 146 |
| 22. Confusion and Coma | 155 |
| 23. Meningoencephalitis | 163 |
| 24. Cerebrovascular Stroke | 171 |
| 25. Miscellaneous | 185 |
| *Abbreviations* | 189 |
| *Index* | 193 |

# Introduction

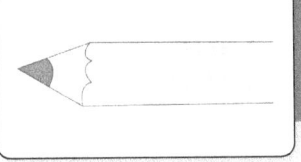

Neurology is a fascinating branch of medicine, very analytical and very interesting. There are several myths regarding clinical neurology.

**Myth 1—Neurology is a very difficult subject to understand**

Majority of doctors are not comfortable dealing with a patient having a neurological problem. The reason for fear is due to inadequate training in basic clinical approach to Neurology.

The truth is that among all the medical topics, neurology is the easiest, where 2+2 is almost equal to 4. The exact anatomical localization can be derived from the history and physical findings, which can now be confirmed by various investigations. For example, if a patient has sensory and motor symptoms in right lower limb it is due to radiculopathy/plexopathy on the right side; on the other hand if sensory symptoms are present in right lower limb and motor symptoms in left lower limb then the lesion is in left half of the thoracic spinal cord. In case of foot drop, if ankle jerk is absent then it is L5 radiculopathy, if ankle jerk is intact then it is lateral popliteal nerve palsy! It is simple and easy!

**Myth 2—Neurological examination is elaborate and time consuming**

Diagnosis can be easily arrived at by history taking (80%), examination, (10%) and basic investigations (5%). Only the remaining 5% is diagnosed by high-tech investigations. This holds true even today, in spite of a plethora of investigations. The neurological examination need not be elaborate and time consuming in all patients. Focused neurological examination, i.e. focusing on that part of neurological examination which confirms the provisional diagnosis after *obtaining the history* is all that is required. This requires a working diagnosis at the end of history.

**Myth 3—Why waste time on clinical diagnosis, when there are enough investigations to clinch the diagnosis**

With the exponential growth of diagnostic facilities like imaging (CT, MR), EEG, ENMG, and other advanced laboratory techniques, one may start believing that these expensive investigations will give the correct diagnosis. However, it is just the opposite. When investigations are used with no clinical diagnosis it leads to wrong diagnosis and treatment; investigations without a clinical diagnosis is like wearing a tie without clothes!!.

When I trained in clinical neurology such imaging techniques were not available. Now I am happy to note that these imaging techniques only confirm the clinical skills which I had acquired earlier by precisely localizing the anatomical site of the lesion.

Any investigation has to be interpreted on the strength of the clinical diagnosis, as the investigation report by itself may be incidental or non-contributory to the diagnosis or even misleading, e.g. the MR lumbar spine of a patient with spastic paraparesis shows a disc prolapse at L 4-5; obviously the radiological findings are irrelevant to the clinical diagnosis. Spasticity is due to upper motor neuron lesion in spinal cord and spinal cord ends at lower border of L1 Vertebra even in 2017!! And hence at L 4-5 there is no spinal cord!. Another example is that of a patient with non-epileptic attack disorder (psychogenic seizures) who may have non-specific EEG changes. One should not diagnose it as epilepsy based only on the EEG report.

There are many incidental findings in imaging of the brain like lacunar infarcts, calcified granuloma, cerebral atrophy and even small incidental meningiomas! MR of cervical or lumbar region after the age of 50 years may show disc prolapse, sometimes even indentation of spinal cord or roots; however the symptoms may not be due to what is seen in the image!. This may lead to wrong diagnosis and wrong surgical treatment. It is only clinical diagnosis which will tell us whether these findings are relevant or not. It should always be 'think first and investigate later' and not the reverse which unfortunately is what is being practiced today. Relying heavily on scans for diagnosis leads to 'Scan is normal and so the person is normal too' philosophy.

It should be remembered that any investigation provides the report of the observer, e.g. a Radiologist. The clinician has the distinct advantage and responsibility of evaluating the patient as a whole, whereas the investigations will only look at the patient through 'a hole'! A clinician is like a Master Chef who has access to all the ingredients—history, onset, evolution, clinical findings and a host of investigations starting from hematological, biochemical, imaging, electrophysiological and so on. It is up to the master chef to use these ingredients and intelligently mix it up to produce a final diagnosis!

Even today, common neurological diseases have only clinical diagnosis as the final diagnosis, with no confirmatory investigations or tests available! Take for example all varieties of headache (including migraine and cluster headache), epilepsy, the whole range of movement disorders starting from tremors, Parkinson's disease to chorea, athetosis and dystonia and the emerging epidemic disorder of dementia. These conditions are diagnosed only clinically, as there are no investigations to confirm the diagnosis.

**Myth 4—Neurological diagnosis is a futile exercise, as most of these conditions have no treatment**

With advances in the field of neurology, the management of common diseases like epilepsy, stroke, Parkinson's disease, neuro infections and multiple sclerosis have vastly improved to benefit the patients.

| Myths | Facts |
| --- | --- |
| 1. Difficult to understand and practice | Most analytical, easy to practice provided one follows a disciplined approach |
| 2. Hi-tech investigations will give diagnosis so why waste time on elaborate history and neurological examination. | Many investigations provide incidental, non-relevant and non-contributory findings |
| 3. Neurological examination is lengthy and time consuming | Focused neurological examination focusing on the relevant part as determined at the end of history taking, is informative |
| 4. Most diseases have no treatment | Recent advances have offered treatment for various diseases like stroke, Parkinson's disease, epilepsy, neuro infection, multiple sclerosis, etc. |

**Over Investigating the Patient**

It is now well understood by laymen, patients and doctors that healthcare has become a 'healthcare industry'. It is no more a healthy care! The industry is run by corporate houses and is managed by management experts whose goal is to increase the profits. This leads to patients being asked to undergo unnecessary and expensive investigations. It is heartening to note that this factor is being addressed by the medical community in various countries. In USA, the 'choosing wisely campaign' has been started wherein the emphasis is on recommendation for performing only necessary investigations. For example, the American Academy of Neurology recommends not to perform EEG for headache and imaging of carotid arteries for simple syncope. In India, recently, a group of doctors from AIIMS, New Delhi founded the Society for Less Investigative Medicine (SLIM) to educate patients and doctors about the evils of excessive investigations.

The words of Aldous Huxley who said that 'Medical science has made such tremendous progress that there is hardly a healthy human left', is apt here.

## DON'T TREAT THE DISEASE—TREAT THE PATIENT WITH THE DISEASE

Diagnosis does not automatically mean treatment. For example, a 50-year-old man consulted a physician for fever and the brilliant physician observed that he was not moving the left upper limb as smoothly as the right. The doctor diagnosed it as Parkinson's disease and started him on L-dopa. Now the diagnosis is very correct but there is no medicine to cure Parkinson's disease nor to slow the progress of the disease. Only symptomatic treatment is available for tremor and rigidity. If the patient's daily activities are not affected then there is no need to start any treatment! On the contrary, starting L-dopa so early, may show deleterious side effects later on, when the drug is required. If a patient consults a doctor for mild tremors of hands – 'essential tremors'—but if he is able to carry on all his activities unaffected then there is no need to put him on any medication because the medication will only suppress the tremors, not cure the disease. Hence, why suppress the tremors with medication if it is not bothering the patient? *Do not treat the disease, treat the patient with the disease.*

## PRESCRIBE BARE ESSENTIAL DRUGS

Very commonly I see a long list of medicines being prescribed to patients and many a times when such a patient consults me I take off the unnecessary medications. Such medications are a burden to the patient in terms of the cost. There are many drugs of dubious value in the market like cerebrolysin, citicoline ginkgo biloba, piracetam, pyritinol, etc. A variety of pills with A to Z vitamins, minerals, etc. which too have no clinical value are also available in abundance! It is criminal to prescribe such expensive drugs to a patient who has no money for two square meals a day!

Even when a drug is necessary, one should look into prescribing a cost effective drug, for example, in the management of epilepsy when medicines have to be taken for a period of two to five years, where is the need to prescribe the expensive levetiracetam when less costly drugs like phenytoin or carbamazepine which are equally effective in treating the condition are available. I have seen auto rickshaw drivers and labourers being prescribed such expensive medicines who lament that they have to cut down on their food to meet the drug expenses. Here again effective generic drugs should be prescribed rather than expensive branded drugs.

To sum it up, before prescribing a medicine it is important to pause and think as to whether the drugs are necessary, if so depending upon the economic condition of the patient the less expensive drug should be prescribed.

The following are the general principles in clinical neurology.
a.  It is not taking down the history as told by the patient but eliciting the history with more detailed relevant questioning that is important. Medical history taking is an art which has to be learnt and practiced. The patient will obviously emphasize on the most disabling symptoms, but for a clinician even a subtle symptom may give a clue to a diagnosis.
b.  Any neurological disability should be assessed by its impact on the activities of daily living, e.g. a patient complains of giddiness and is unstable while walking and yet can run and catch a bus; obviously this is a non- disabling symptom as compared to a person whose imbalance requires support even within the house.
c.  The adage 'tell me who your friend is and I will tell you who you are' also applies to the anatomical localization. If a person has spastic quadriparesis with a 'symptom friend' of dysarthria then the localization is to the brainstem and requires imaging of the brain, while in spastic quadriparesis with severe neck pain the localization is to the cervical cord.
d.  The disease is dynamic and evolution of the disease is like watching a striptease show! If you are too early a lot is left for guessing and imagination and if you come in much later the diagnosis is obvious. For example, a patient presents with facial palsy—the immediate diagnosis is Bell's palsy. Three days later he develops proximal muscle weakness at which time the diagnosis of GB syndrome can easily be made. That diagnosis cannot be made at the time of first consultation!
e.  To minimize time and be precise, focused neurological examination is very helpful, i.e. focusing on that part of the nervous system as assessed by the history.
f.  Random investigations do not help in diagnosis. Infact, the incidental findings may be misleading. Hence, investigations should be done only after appropriate anatomical diagnosis. For example, in a person with proximal muscle weakness of lower limb, generally an MR of lumbar spine is done. However, if the clinical diagnosis is polymyositis, then CK and ENMG are required, not MR of lumbar spine.
g.  Diagnosis does not mean immediate prescription and treatment. For example, early Parkinson's disease with mild rigidity of left upper limb (in right handed individuals) not affecting the daily activities does not need any treatment. While the same mild rigidity in the right handed which affects signature of an executive requires appropriate therapy. Every symptom has to be assessed by the disability for activities of daily living.
h.  Review your own diagnosis also; not only that of others!

# CHAPTER 2

# History

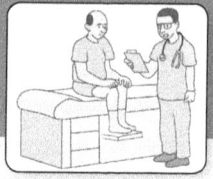

## HOW TO OBTAIN HISTORY?

History is important in all spheres of life, whether it is recruiting a person for a job, or choosing a spouse, we all depend on the history. Similarly in clinical medicine the history of illness (onset, progression, duration), personal history, past history, family history are all important.

History taking is an art which has to be learnt and practiced by observing the seniors and has to be developed over a period of time.

History tells us what the problem is and physical examination where the problem is.

One should have eye to eye contact with the patient while eliciting the history and while conversing with the patient because the patient should know that you are attentive and interested to hear his story. It is a common complaint by patients, that the doctors are busy multitasking—answering phone calls, instructing the assistants, looking at the smart phone, I-pad, computer, etc. and hardly listen to them. Many of the stress-related symptoms can be reduced if the patient knows that the doctor is listening carefully with undivided attention.

Many of the litigations are due to non-communication with the concerned persons. Before I explain in detail the nature of the illness and the condition of the patient, I make sure that I am talking to the first degree relatives (spouse, son, daughter) and not to a cousin who has just landed from USA or from some other city! This is to avoid a situation where the immediate relative will complain that the doctor has not explained the seriousness of the illness.

History taking today has become more difficult as patients no longer talk about the symptoms, but about the diagnosis or findings of the investigations. For example, a patient may say "Doctor, I have cervical spondylosis" or "I have L4-L5 disc prolapse". Similarly, instead of complaining of episodic giddiness, they start off by saying that the "MR brain showed several lacunar infarcts"!

Often, patients only talk about their neurological symptoms to the neurologists without mentioning other symptoms like chest pain and palpitation for which they have been extensively investigated and found to be normal. So, I keep asking them "any other symptom?" and they say "No". But when specifically asked — "did you have chest pain, palpitation, acidity", they say "yes, but all investigations were normal". When confronted as to why they did not mention such symptoms, the reply is that since it does not deal with my speciality, they felt it was not important to mention them! On the contrary when my diagnosis is tension headache, symptoms like chest pain, palpitation and acidity strengthens the diagnosis. Detailed history gives more information for the diagnosis.

When patients are not attentive to my questions I remind them that my diagnosis depends on their observations and if they give wrong information I will offer a wrong diagnosis! This is to make them understand that a doctor is asking so many questions to help them and not to while away the time! Patients usually think that a scan or examination by doctor is enough to make a diagnosis so why is he asking so many questions?

## MAKE SURE THE HISTORY IS BEING GIVEN BY A PERSON WHO HAS WITNESSED IT

It is interesting to note that we get a very descriptive history from the person who has not observed the event! The patient's son who is living in USA comes for a brief visit and brings his dad for consultation and gives a fantastic history—particularly with reference to onset and progress of the disease even though he is unaware of it. The first question I ask is "do you live with the patient?" The children may be living in the same city, but independently, in which case the spouse or the caregiver has to be questioned for detailed information.

History not only from the patient but from people living and working with the patient will be necessary to elicit the changes in personality, memory issues, hallucinations, etc. as in dementia.

Epilepsy is entirely a clinical diagnosis and it is necessary to get an eyewitness account of the event.

The history given by a person who brings the patient to the hospital runs like this "she was sitting on a chair, suddenly she felt giddy and fell down unconscious and we shifted her to the hospital". When a more detailed history is obtained from the person who was present at that time, the story runs like this "she fell off the chair, had seizures and regained consciousness but was confused, could walk with support to the car and she was shifted to the hospital". Now the history is totally different and is suggestive of seizure disorder.

Usually the relatives or the attendants of the patient will say "nothing has happened" "she just felt giddy as she did not have breakfast". Even though she had a seizure, they just want to reassure. Then I pin them down saying "please describe what you have seen to help the patient get a proper diagnosis".

Chief complaints are the starting point for further active questioning, probing into the onset of symptoms, duration, and progression. The history also assists in anatomical localization, e.g. patient complains of weakness of right hand to mix food, write, buttoning. The anatomical localization can be at the level of muscle, peripheral nerve, plexus, spinal cord or contra lateral cerebral hemisphere. Enquiring about alteration of speech will localize the lesion to cerebral hemisphere. Patients will only complain what causes the disability, however eliciting a few more symptoms will help the clinician for proper diagnosis. The best way to elicit is to run through the activities of daily living.

## ACTIVITIES OF DAILY LIVING (ADL)

One need not be a neurologist to know the activities of daily living like getting out of the bed, using the toilet, brushing, shaving, washing face, eating breakfast, bathing, dressing up and going to work. One has to ask whether all these activities can be done normally as before, can be done with some difficulty, done with assistance, cannot be done at all. This is a very important parameter to assess the disability due to illness and evolution of the illness, on which depends the clinical diagnosis. An acute onset with recovery happens in vascular disorders and seizure disorders. Transient loss of consciousness with total recovery can be seizure, syncope, hypoglycemia or transient ischemic attack (TIA). Relentlessly progressive disease for more than a year is likely to be benign compressive pathology (e.g. cervical spondylotic myelopathy) or degenerative disease.

A patient may complain of continuous giddiness of two weeks duration. Ask how it affects daily activities? If the patient is able to carry out all the daily activities unaffected, including walking briskly to catch the bus, then obviously it is psychogenic. If the giddiness is briefly incapacitating, then it is an organic condition.

While a patient may just say weakness of right arm, it is necessary to probe further and find out what activities are affected, e.g. mixing food, writing (distal muscles), combing hair, brushing (proximal muscles), associated difficulty in talking (cerebral localization).

With reference to evolution of the illness — whether it is static, improving or worsening — again history is important. Detailed questioning about the activities of daily living gives a clue to the progress of the illness, e.g. in a person who requires assistance to walk in the first week of illness, but is able to walk unaided in the third week, it is an improvement, but in a person who could mix food in the first week of illness and is unable to do so in the later weeks, it is worsening of the illness. Activities of daily living like brushing teeth, bathing, dressing, eating, etc. are markers for following the progress of the disease — improving, status quo or deteriorating. Traditional neurological findings of power of muscles like 2/5, 3/5 are far less informative than saying "unable to mix food" to "able to mix food".

## PAST HISTORY

Of course, history of hypertension, diabetes, hypothyroid, etc. have to be elicited. What is also important is "drug history". Use of tranquilizers, ayurvedic, homeopathy, and alternative medicines may have an impact on the present illness. All "pathies" are to be explored—homeopathy, naturopathy, allopathy.

Past medical history with details of symptoms is important and not the diagnostic label. For example, if a patient says "Doctor I had a stroke 2 years ago," he may mean paralysis or seizure or unconsciousness.

A question like "did you have similar illness in the past", elicits an instantaneous reply "No". I tell them please think, take time and answer, as some illnesses which have recurrent episodes like severe migraine headaches may not require an investigation whereas a first time severe headache needs investigation.

*Personal history* regarding the habits addressing smoking or tobacco chewing, alcohol, recreational drugs, not necessarily at present but even in the past is important. When I ask the patient "do you smoke or drink", the immediate answer is "No". But when I ask "not now, what about in the past?" the reply is "I gave it up two years ago!" but the wife rebuts that he did smoke and drink for 20 years and stopped it only since the past two months!

*Family history* of similar illness is an important marker for heredodegenerative disorders, e.g. a person who has cerebellar ataxia of two months duration and has similar illness in the family does not need elaborate investigations and also the prognosis is totally different. However eliciting family history is another ball game! Earlier a family consisted of 6-10 children and an informative family history was available. Now a days it is only one or two children and often they live in different countries and are unaware of subtle symptoms in the other sibling. It is much more difficult to get information from the families of cousins, uncles and aunts as intra-family communications have become sparse! When asked, "does anybody in your family have a similar illness", there will be an immediate and instantaneous answer "No". However when further questioned about the number of family members and when was the last time they met the answer is "not for several years". When I question the patient, whether any of his relatives are aware of his illness, he says no. Then how do you expect to know similar illness in other family members.

## INADEQUATE HISOTRY

Often we mention that "history is inadequate" which is the fault of the doctor and not the patient. May be another visit, when both the patient and the doctor are relatively free and fresh, is required to obtain more history. The best way to solve a diagnostic dilemma is not by ordering more sophisticated investigations but making efforts to get proper history. Try to obtain information from members living with the patient and colleagues working with him.

## WHY DOES THE DIAGNOSIS CHANGE WITH TIME?

The process of the disease is often dynamic — progressing over a period of few days to weeks or months. So naturally the clinician who sees the patient during the later part of illness is at an advantage to make a better diagnosis! The disease unfolds gradually and it is like watching a striptease show, the one who enters the show early has to have a lot of imagination whereas the one who enters last sees everything!

*Case History*: A 72-year-old male presented with history of intermittent twitching of left side of face of 2 days duration. Clinical diagnosis was left partial motor seizures involving the face. CT head scan showed a small ring enhancing lesion in the right frontal lobe—probable solitary cysticercus lesion—which was treated with antiepileptic drugs Carbamazepine and Albendazole. On the fourth day he developed left faciobrachial paresis which warranted a repeat scan. The MR brain—plain and contrast—showed increase in the size of the lesion, which was now multiloculated with extensive perilesional edema suggestive of pyogenic abscess, which was confirmed at surgery.

Here the disease unfolded over a few days and the diagnosis changed when new symptoms and signs were added. Do not blame the previous doctor for wrong diagnosis; he only entered the scene at the wrong time!

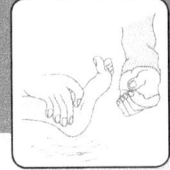 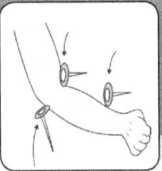

# CHAPTER 3
# Neurological Examination

Contrary to the perception that neurological examination is time-consuming and laborious, it can be assessed quickly and comprehensively. The structured neurological examination consists of higher functions, viz. speech, optic fundi, cranial nerves, motor system, sensory system, cerebellar features, gait, skull and spine. How can we do this in a short span of 10 minutes?

The neurological examination need not always be elaborate. It can be a *focused neurological examination* which means "focus on the symptoms". If the patient has difficulty in walking and no symptoms in upper limbs the focused neurological examination is on the lower limbs. It becomes very easy to make a quick diagnosis if the patient's symptoms are better understood by asking him to do that activity which is bothering him, e.g. a person with difficulty in writing should be asked to write in front of you to see what the difficulty is due to — is it a tremor, or dystonia; if the patient has difficulty in walking he should be asked to walk and his gait should be observed which will give the diagnosis; the time spent on examining the patient on the couch should be lessened!

The neurological examination starts by observing the way the patient enters the consulting room—the gait, the arm swing.

## HIGHER FUNCTIONS

As the history is being elicited one can simultaneously grasp the higher functions like memory, orientation and alertness. However when a specific examination is required as in dementia/acute confusion, a bedside screening test for higher mental function is necessary. This testing requires four frontal lobes—two of the examiner's (he should be attentive while performing this test) and two of the patient's (he should be attentive and cooperative while answering the questions). The test measures alertness, orientation to time, place and persons, attention and concentration (which includes digit span and counting numbers backwards) and memory (immediate and past). Similarly as the patient is talking, one can observe whether the speech is normal or abnormal; then go on to optic fundus examination without dilating the pupil.

## CRANIAL NERVES

Olfactory nerve is examined when required.

Vision test, by closing one eye at a time for distant and near vision, should be conducted. Field defects at the bed side can be assessed by "confrontation test" by asking the patient to sit at a distance of 18", close the right eye of the patient and left eye of the examiner and bring the tip of the pen from periphery to central in horizontal and then in vertical direction. Repeat with closure of patient's, left eye and right eye of the examiner.

*Examination of ocular movements*: Stand in front of the patient at a distance of 3 feet, hold a pen in your hand and ask the patient to look at the tip of the pen, observe the ocular movements while moving the pen in either direction—horizontally and vertically; look for disconjugate movement with or without diplopia. With diplopia there are two images and the outer image belongs to paretic muscle. These are called "following" or "slow" movements. To test for "saccades" or fast movements ask the patient to follow the tip of the pen which is moved fast in both horizontal and vertical direction.

V motor examination is done by clenching of the teeth and palpation of temporalis and masseter muscles. Sensory V nerve examination is by cotton touch, pin and corneal reflex. For VII nerve examination, as the patient is talking, deviation of the angle of the mouth should be observed. The VII nerve examination consists of lifting of the eye brows, tight closure of the eyelids against resistance, blowing of the cheek and showing of the teeth with angle of the mouth drawn outwards. Hearing can be tested by simple rubbing of the thumb and index near the external ears and comparing both the ears. Asking the patient to open the mouth and say "Ah" will demonstrate the soft palate movement, gag reflex can be observed by touching the posterior pharyngeal wall with cotton swab. For XI cranial nerve examination, the patient is asked to shrug his shoulders and turn his head laterally and bend forward against resistance offered by the examiner. For XII cranial nerve the patient is asked to move his tongue from side to side and up and down.

Gag reflex, corneal reflex when absent bilaterally is not necessarily pathologic, while unilateral absence is pathological.

## MOTOR SYSTEM

Structured motor system examination consists of nutrition, tone, power, coordination, abnormal movement and elicitation of reflexes *in that order*. Global wasting of all four limbs is due to systemic conditions like chronic infection (TB), malignancy and malnutrition. The motor power is marginally and symmetrically reduced. However neurological wasting, is asymmetric and the wasted muscle shows decreased motor power. The examination of the tone will tell whether there is stiffness [Upper motor neuron (UMN), extrapyramidal disorder] or reduced tone as in lower motor neuron and muscle diseases. The tone has to be elicited for groups of muscles in each joint like wrist, elbow, knee and ankle and the passive resistance offered should be observed. To test tone, the patient should be completely relaxed. Often patients are tense and resist passive movement or try to help the doctor by actively moving the limb! The best way is to keep the patient engaged by talking, so that adequate relaxation of muscles is possible. The examination of the power of the muscles follows the tone because if there is stiffness of the muscles as a result of rigidity or spasticity the full range of movement of joint is not possible, then the interpretation should be "cannot assess the power because of rigidity" and it should not be concluded that power is 1/5! Coordination is tested following the examination for tone and power. If the patient has gross spasticity, or significant motor weakness, coordination is affected. If tone and power are normal and yet there is incoordination then it reflects cerebellar system involvement. Abnormal movements can be seen in the form of fasciculations, which, when present indicate degenerating anterior horn cell disease, or irritation of motor root, occasionally due to motor peripheral nerve. Tendon reflexes again may be difficult to elicit if there is too much spasticity or rigidity. This is the importance of *following structured motor system examination.*

## Motor System Examination of Upper Limbs

Examine the patient in sitting position for tone and power by gripping the hand and flexion and extension at elbow; ask the patient to keep both the arms stretched in front, maintaining the posture; test for other movements at shoulder; finger nose test with either limbs and rapid alternate movement of the hands.

Motor system examination of the lower limbs is quite easy. Ask the patient to walk up and down, first normally and then with a quicker pace which will give an idea of stiffness of limbs as in spasticity, motor weakness if dragging one limb as in hemiparesis, waddling gait in proximal muscle weakness and short shuffling gait in Parkinson's disease. If there is instability while making about turn, it may point to early cerebellar involvement. Next ask the patient to walk on the heels which tests the dorsiflexors of the ankle (L5) and then to walk on toes which tests plantarflexors (S1) of the ankle. Next the patient should be asked to walk in a straight line keeping one foot in front of the other to test for gait coordination. Patient should then be asked to sit on the floor and get up to test for proximal muscle weakness, stand on one leg to assess the motor power. If the patient is able to hop on one leg at a time, then it shows that everything is fine with the lower limbs. Lastly the patient is asked to lie down on the couch, and reflexes are elicited. Time and again emphasis is placed on tendon reflexes and plantar reflexes—both these findings have relevance *only* if some *neurological signs are observed in the motor system.* Remember the examination order for motor system.

## SENSORY EXAMINATION

Sensory examination is required only if there is a lead to sensory impairment. Sensory examination requires four frontal lobes, two of the patient's and two of the examiner's; both patient and doctor should be alert and attentive! Sensory examination is done with cotton, pin and appropriate tuning fork. Often the patient continues to say "yes" even when not touched with the pin! Then I tell them that they should be attentive as my diagnosis depends on their observation, e.g. to differentiate acute transverse myelitis from Guillain-barre syndrome presence or absence of sensory is crucial.

Next, one should turn the patient and look for any tenderness, deformities of the spine. Also carefully look for perianal anesthesia for diagnosis of cauda equina syndrome. This completes the quick out patient department (OPD) focused neurological examination.

## FOLLOW-UP

During follow-up the patient and the physician are interested in restoration of activities of daily living rather than mere notings such as 2/5, 4/5 power. Making notes such as "difficulty in getting up from squatting position, but not from the chair" is more meaningful both to the patient and the doctor than saying 2/5 or 3+/5. "Difficulty in mixing food, later able to mix food" is a more meaningful interpretation than 3/5 to 5/5 motor power!

At the end of the examination the neurological diagnosis can be divided into the following 4 steps:
1. Neurological deficit/dysfunction
2. Anatomical localization
3. Pathological diagnosis
4. Etiological diagnosis

If one follows these steps diligently one can make a fairly accurate clinical diagnosis for most of the day to day neurological problems.

*Let me elaborate;*

### Step 1: Neurological Deficit/Dysfunction

At the end of history taking one gets a fair idea of the patient's problem. For example, if the history is difficulty to walk and difficulty to pass urine a focused neurological examination shows paraparesis with sensory impairment below D6 level.

**Neurological Deficit**
a. Paraparesis due to upper motor neuron lesion
b. Sensory level at D6
c. Bladder dysfunction from history

d. If at the time of examination the patient has paraplegia, but the history clearly shows asymmetric onset, this should be noted down in step 1 as "compressive lesions present in asymmetric fashion". Paraparesis has 3 components—motor, sensory and bladder. All three should be assessed. Before proceeding to step 2, confirm whether all symptoms in history have been explained in step 1.

### Step 2: Anatomical Localization

This is extremely important to determine the type of investigations to be done and the area to be investigated. For example, if the patient's problem is difficulty in walking due to spastic paraparesis and examination also shows brisk reflexes in upper limb with weakness of triceps then the anatomical localization will be lower cervical cord and the imaging should be MR cervical cord even though the patient has only symptoms in lower limb. In a situation like this, one should spend more time in examining the upper limb for subtle signs for proper anatomical localization. Often patients with UMN paraparesis are made to undergo MR lumbosacral spine for difficulty in walking ! forgetting that spinal cord ends at L1 level. So how can UMN paraparesis occur with lumbosacral area pathology?

The second point is that for anatomical localization the adage "tell me who your friends are and I will tell you who you are" is much suited. For example, if a patient has sensory symptoms in the right hand and also has difficulty in walking due to stiffness of limbs, the localization is to the cervical cord. Stiffness is an UMN lesion and it has to be in the spinal cord while the sensory cervical cord. Stiffness symptoms can be peripheral or in the cervical cord. The common factor here is the cervical cord and so the anatomical localization for sensory symptoms is cervical cord in view of the "friend" corticospinal tract.

Subacute flaccid paraplegia can be due to lower motor neuron (LMN) paralysis (Guillain-barre syndrome) or UMN paralysis (transverse myelitis). If sensory level is at D8/D10, "this friend" helps to localize to spinal cord.

Before proceeding to step 3, make sure that the anatomical localization explains all the neurological deficits. If history of seizures is present, add cerebral localization also in step 2.

### Step 3: Pathological Diagnosis

This takes into account the onset and progress of the illness. Sudden onset of an illness is due to a vascular cause (all varieties of stroke) or traumatic injuries. At the other end of the spectrum is a very chronic disorder, where the illness unfolds over a period of several months or years, such as, degenerative disorders like Alzheimer's dementia, motor neuron disease, muscular dystrophy. One should also consider treatable benign compressive disorders like cervical spondylosis, spinal canal stenosis, meningioma. Diseases evolving over a period of a few days are usually due to infection (e.g. meningitis), demyelination (e.g. multiple sclerosis) and those evolving over a period of several weeks can be due to space occupying lesions (e.g. subdural hematoma, tumors and abscess), toxicity (alcohol), or some deficiency (Vitamin B12). Remember that the pathological diagnosis is at the anatomical site that has been determined in stage 2. For example, if there are more than 2 anatomical sites the space occupying lesion becomes less likely. A person having proximal muscle weakness in upper and lower limbs cannot have compressive lesions on both sides of cervical cord and lumbar region.

### Step 4: Etiological Diagnosis

This is the final diagnosis. If the pathological diagnosis is vascular then the etiological diagnosis would be atherosclerosis or arteritis. Similarly if the space occupying lesion is inflammatory in nature then tuberculosis, fungal, pyogenic possibilities should be considered.

Investigations are of two specific types: (a) investigation for confirming anatomical localization, e.g. magnetic resonance imaging (MRI) spinal cord, MRI brain, Electroneuromyography (ENMG) for peripheral nervous system, (b) investigation for etiological diagnosis, e.g. biopsy, cerebrospinal fluid (CSF) examination.

***Case History:*** A 30-year-female doctor had low backache and difficulty in walking with occasional pain in right lower limb. She also had difficulty to grip the slippers of the right foot of 3 months duration. The treating physician came to the conclusion "low backache with a foot drop = lumbar disc prolapse". An MR lumbosacral spine showed L 4–5 disc prolapse and she was posted for surgery. However neurological examination revealed *spastic foot drop* with exaggerated ankle jerk which clearly shows the presence of an UMN lesion, the vague pain in the back and the right lower limb was because of spasticity.

*Step 1*: Neurological deficit—UMN right lower limb monoparesis
*Step 2*: Anatomical localization—Thoracic spinal cord, right side level—indeterminate as no sensory loss; but upper limbs being normal, below D1 (thoracic spine)
*Step 3*: Pathological diagnosis—subacute progressive—compressive pathology?
*Step 4*: Etiological diagnosis—depends on the investigation.

Investigation for anatomical localization—MR thoracic spine, plain and contrast revealed D6 neurofibroma on right side compressing the spinal cord, which was operated subsequently, and confirmed by histopathology. This clearly shows the importance of anatomical localization and appropriate imaging. Here the L4–5 disc prolapse was incidental.

***Diagnosis:*** Neurofibroma D6 level.

***Case History:*** A 60-year-old woman presented with chronic history of aches and pains of one year duration. The pain started with low back and then spread to the muscles of the thighs, and subsequently progressed to neck and shoulder. Her difficulty in walking was initially diagnosed due to "lumbar spondylosis" and subsequently also "cervical spondylosis". This patient happened to be a doctor's relative who came in with a bundle of CT and MR scans of the lumbar spine, thoracic spine, cervical spine and also of the brain! When asked as to why all these scans were done, she replied that as she was from outstation in case she was asked to do the MR brain she had no time for the same and so had got MR brain too done! Clinical examination revealed distinct proximal muscle weakness, both in lower and upper limbs with preserved reflexes.

*Step 1*: Neurological dysfunction—pain and difficulty in walking due to proximal muscle weakness.

*Step 2*: The anatomical localization is the muscle

*Step 3*: Pathological diagnosis chronic progressive –? Inflammatory (polymyositis)? degenerative (muscular dystrophy) and hence the investigation should be directed to the muscle disease. Investigation of choice to confirm anatomical localization – CK, (3500 iu), EMG

*Step 4*: Investigation for etiological diagnosis—muscle biopsy confirmed chronic polymyositis

**Diagnosis:** Chronic polymyositis.

**Case History:** *Quite often* the final diagnosis is based just on the clinical diagnosis with no confirmatory tests available. A 30-year-old lady came with history of pain in the left side of neck and face of 6 months duration. The history also revealed that the pain was occurring intermittently, worsened by neck muscles becoming stiff. As the stiffness was in the face and neck a host of specialists were consulted. The list of investigations included X-rays, imaging of the brain, cervical spine with the diagnosis of atypical facial pain/functional/trigeminal neuralgia/caries tooth. In fact two teeth from the side of facial pain had been removed! The diagnosis was obvious while talking to the patient as she had involuntary intermittent sustained spasm of the left face and neck muscles.

*Step 1*: Neurological deficit—"cervical dystonia".

*Step 2*: Anatomical localization-basal ganglia, but there is no way to confirm the diagnosis by any investigative procedure! However the correct diagnosis benefited the patient in terms of appropriate management

*Step 3*: Pathological diagnosis—slow progressive? degenerative

**Diagnosis:** Cervical dystonia.

Remember that common neurological disorders, e.g. headache, epilepsy, Parkinson's disease, dementia all are only clinical diagnosis. There are no confirmatory investigations.

**Case History:** A 30-year-old male in good health, developed weakness of right lower limb with difficulty in gripping the slippers and dragging the limb while walking because of stiffness. At this stage the thought process is right lower limb motor weakness due to UMN (in view of history of stiffness in the leg). The anatomical localization would be anywhere in the corticospinal tract from the precentral cortex in the left hemisphere down to thoracic spinal cord through corona radiata internal capsule, cerebral peduncle, brainstem and then ipsilateral corticospinal tract in the spinal cord. The following week he developed right lower limb partial seizures.

*Step 1*: Right lower limb spastic paresis

*Step 2*: Anatomical localization—The friend "right lower limb partial seizures" localizes to contralateral cerebral hemispheres—in motor area.

*Step 3*: Pathological diagnosis—subacute progressive disease—infection (TB)/tumor

*Step 4*: Etiological diagnosis—depends on the investigation reports

*Investigation* of choice to confirm the anatomical localization is MR brain plain and contrast—contrast is required to delineate inflammatory pathology—MR brain showed tumor over left motor strip.

***Diagnosis:*** Glioma left cerebral hemisphere.

## NEUROLOGICAL EXAMINATION IN ICU

In the intensive care unit (ICU) several vital parameters are assessed automatically on the panel which includes blood pressure, pulse, respiration, continuous ECG monitoring, etc. and blood is drawn regularly for a variety of investigations like $PaO_2$, $PCO_2$ metabolic workup, and electrolytes and chest X-ray is repeated every day. However what is missing in the general ICU is neurological evaluation like assessing the level of sensorium with or without painful stimuli, noting down the response of pupils, evidence of neurological deficits like hemiplegia—all these require a human interaction with the patient and not machine recording! Unfortunately in the general ICU these are not properly emphasized. The details are mentioned in Chapter 21.

# CHAPTER 4

# Investigations

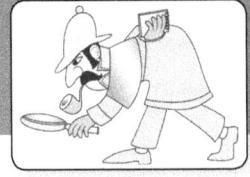

The myth that investigations will provide the diagnosis has to be demystified! In fact investigations may mislead the physician, as there are many incidental observations which are totally non-contributory to the patient's symptoms.

Without clinical localization one blindly asks for CT/MRI scan and follows what is shown in the imaging. Patients with complaints of episodic giddiness are investigated with carotid doppler which shows incidental stenosis and a conclusion is drawn that it is due to cerebrovascular ischemia! The patient is started on unnecessary antiplatelet drugs. The patient unnecessarily starts worrying of developing a stroke.

A sharp wave or a spike wave discharge on the EEG is not a confirmation of epilepsy. The EEG may show changes, which have no specific clinical significance such as an ECG showing nonspecific ST-T changes.

The reasons for doing unnecessary investigations are:
a. The patients themselves insist on getting tests done, especially after browsing through the Internet for information from "Google Guru".
b. In today's world where everybody is racing against time, a cursory history and examination by the doctor leads to unnecessary and inappropriate investigations.
c. The *kickbacks* received by doctors for sending patients to diagnostic centers and also the pressure upon the doctors from the corporate hospital managements to increase their revenue.
d. The increasing legal petitions against doctors which results in practice of "defensive medicine". Doctors order tests not because it is required for the patient but to protect themselves against any future legal problems.
e. The gradual deterioration in clinical diagnosis thus relying more and more on investigations.

Unnecessary investigations not only adds to the cost, but also leads to over diagnosis or wrong diagnosis leading to more tests being done thus wasting the patient's time and money and ultimately not being of any help to the patient!

Medical investigations are expensive and increase the healthcare costs. In the US and the UK it is observed that more than 20% of medical investigations are unnecessary. "Choose wisely" campaign was launched in the US in 2012 against unnecessary medical investigations and treatment, which was followed by similar campaigns in the UK, Australia, Japan and 12 other countries.

On similar lines, the Society for Less Investigative Medicine (SLIM) founded by Dr Balram Bhargava and his colleagues in 2014 addresses this growing problem in our country too. The aim is to provide medical practitioners with guidelines for investigations.

## WHEN SHOULD YOU ASK FOR AN INVESTIGATION?

Before you write for an investigation, ask yourself whether it helps in:
a. Diagnosis
b. Management.

Like focused neurological examination, investigations too can be focused, e.g. Investigation to (a) confirm the anatomical localization. If the localization is to the cervical cord, an MR imaging of the cervical spine needs to be done; if the localization is to peripheral nerves, nerve conduction studies need to be done; if it is muscle disease then an EMG needs to be done. The other focused investigation is (b) for etiological diagnosis, e.g. if the diagnosis is herpes simplex encephalitis then an MR brain is suggested for anatomical confirmation and HSV, PCR of CSF for etiological diagnosis.

There are many investigations which are done as "routine" even though it has no bearing on the diagnosis or management of the illness. Apart from being a financial burden on the patient, it is also cumbersome to undergo the investigation. For example, if a long standing diabetic patient complains of burning paresthesia, distally, in both lower limbs with evidence of decreased cotton and pin sensations and absence of ankle jerk, the clinical diagnosis is diabetic peripheral neuropathy and asking for nerve conduction studies is unnecessary and wasteful. Here, the investigation is not going to change the diagnosis or management. In fact, nerve conduction study may be normal if a few large myelinated fibers are intact! So if the report is normal, it is not going to change the clinical diagnosis and if the report is abnormal it is not going to add anything to the clinical diagnosis!

Take another example of a patient admitted with dense right hemiplegia of two days duration. CT scan shows an infarct in the left cerebral hemisphere. Asking for an MR brain in this patient is superfluous. MR will only show more details about the infarct, which is not going to change the diagnosis or the management. Often I see that apart from MR, "routine" carotid Doppler studies are carried out. Carotid Doppler study is done to identify significant stenosis (more than 70%) in the appropriate artery (left internal carotid artery stenosis in a patient who has right hemiplegia) so that carotid intervention (carotid stenting or carotid endarterectomy) can be done to prevent another stroke, *after* meaningful recovery from present stroke.

Similarly MR brain is totally unnecessary in patients with Parkinson's disease, absence epilepsy and juvenile myoclonic epilepsy.

## INVESTIGATIONS AND INDICATIONS

### IMAGING (CT/MR)

Computed tomography and MR imaging of brain and spinal cord have phenomenal impact in diagnosis and management of neurological disorders. *However it does not replace the basic clinical diagnosis.* Image findings have to be correlated with clinical diagnosis. There are many incidental findings in MR imaging which have no clinical relevance.

### CT Head Scan

**Advantages:** Less expensive; easily available in most towns and cities. It takes only a few minutes to do the scan and is thus useful for patients who are uncooperative and restless (Fig. 4.1).

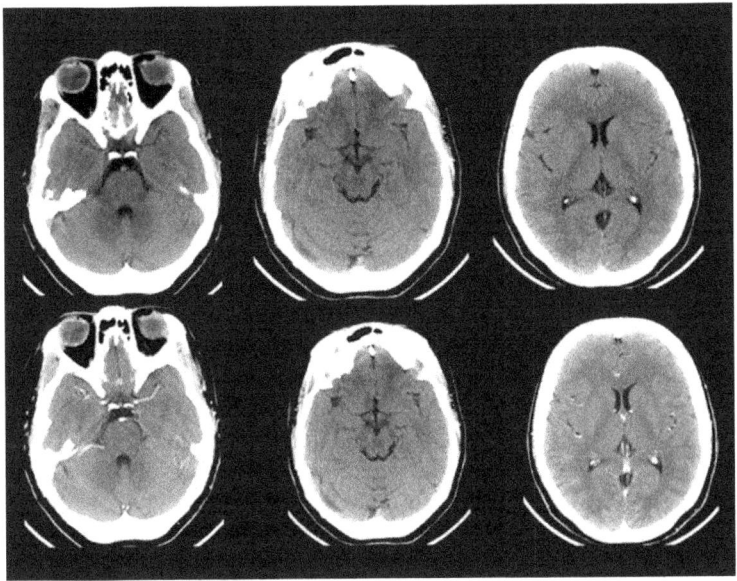

**Fig. 4.1:** CT head scan normal. (Upper row: Plain; lower row: Contrast).

Delineates blood, bone and calcified lesions well. Hence it is an investigation of choice in head injury as the skull bones are clearly defined; shows all the intra cranial bleeds (subdural, subarachnoid, intracerebral), skull vault fractures.

**Disadvantage:** Details of soft tissue—the brain—is not well-visualized (e.g. demyelinating plaques, lacunar infarcts) and exposure to radiation.

CT spine—Useful for bony lesions.

## MR Brain

**Advantages:** Excellent visualization of soft tissue abnormality (Figs. 4.2 and 4.3), e.g. demyelinating plaques, lacunar infarcts, developmental cortical anomalies and medial temporal sclerosis.

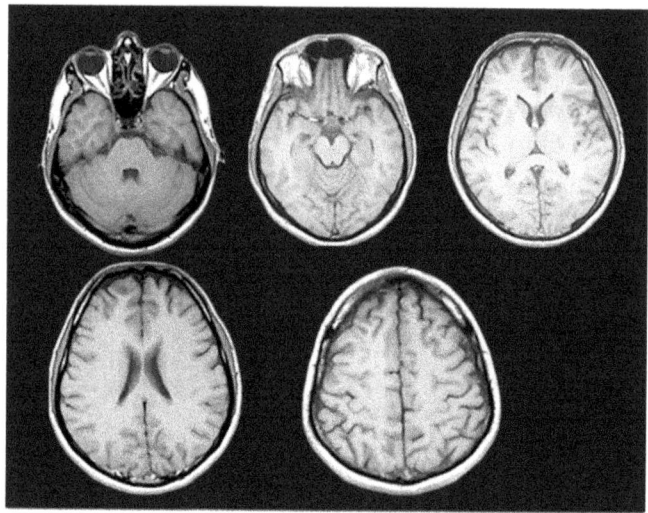

**Fig. 4.2:** MR brain—Normal (axial).

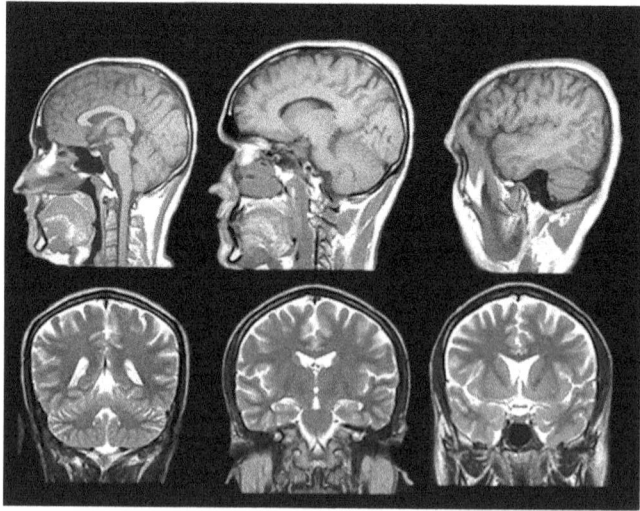

**Fig. 4.3:** MR brain—normal (sagittal, coronal).

**Disadvantages:** Expensive, available only in big cities and takes a longer time to perform; bone lesions and fractures as in head injury not as clearly seen as in CT; proper clinical diagnosis required to select the specific MR sequence (e.g. MR venogram done only when cerebral venous thrombosis is suspected clinically).

**MR Spine:** Visualization of intrinsic and extrinsic cord structures, vertebral column (Figs. 4.4 and 4.5).

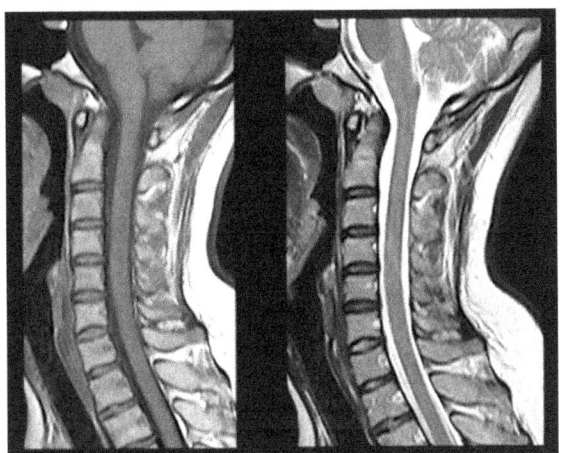

Fig. 4.4: MR cervical spine—normal.

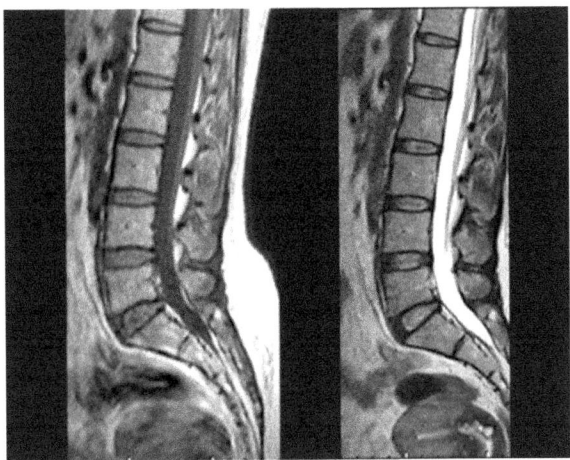

Fig. 4.5: MR lumbar spine—normal.

Differentiating features between CT and MR are shown in Table 4.1.

Table 4.1: Differentiating features between CT and MR.

| | CT | MR |
|---|---|---|
| Cost | ₹ 3,200–3,500 | ₹ 7,000–8,000 |
| Time taken to perform | 5 minutes<br>Useful in restless uncooperative patients | 15–30 minutes<br>Requires cooperation of patient to avoid artifacts |
| X-radiation | Typically 2 millisieverts (mSv) approximately equivalent to 20 chest X-rays | Nil |
| Availability | Even in small towns | Big towns, cities |
| Claustrophobia | Nil | Frequent |
| Imaging of bone, blood calcification | Excellent | Moderate |
| Imaging of soft tissue (brain, spinal cord) | Poor | Excellent |
| Imaging for | Structural (anatomical) abnormality | Greater detail of structural and also functional abnormalities |
| Clinical diagnosis will help to select the variety of imaging | Not necessary | Yes |
| In pregnancy | Not advisable | Yes |
| Metal implant in patient | Can be done | Metal artifacts distort picture |
| Cardiac pacemaker in patient | Can be done | Contraindicated |
| Contrast agent | Nephrotoxic—hence cannot be performed in patients with renal dysfunction | Used in small volume in patients with renal dysfunction and hence side-effects are very few |

## HOW DO YOU WRITE A REQUEST FOR AN MR SCAN?

Quite often the investigation request just mentions the name, viz. "MR brain" or "MR spine." It is necessary to give a brief history and clinical diagnosis and what you are looking for in the imaging. This will help the radiologist to try and answer your query. MR scan of the brain is not akin to ordering a chest X-ray as advances in MR imaging have brought out several techniques addressing different issues—venogram for delineating the venous system, angiogram for intracranial vasculature, diffusion weighted sequences to identify acute ischemic stroke, MR spectroscopy to look into the chemical components of the lesion, MR tractography for viewing white matter. These are in addition to the standard MR sequences of T1, T2, FLAIR images. For example, if clinically D4 level paraparesis is suspected then it should be mentioned with a request to focus on D4 level, as any minor imaging abnormalities like a small demyelinating plaque can be picked up, which may be missed in the "aerial view" image of spine from vertex to coccyx! If the clinical diagnosis is stroke, it should be mentioned in the request form so that DWI and ADC sequences will be done which is specific for acute and subacute infarcts.

Whenever an inflammatory (tuberculoma, cysticercosis, abscess) or vascular (AVM, angioma) lesion is suspected, a contrast must be performed. There is a tendency to think that plain MR will give adequate information, hence why waste money on the expensive contrast material. The contrast seeps whenever a blood brain barrier is broken, or the lesion is vascular.

Both CT and MR visualize the "structural" abnormalities of the brain and spinal cord. In addition MR brain is also used to study "functional" abnormalities. Common clinical indications for imaging are mentioned in Table 4.2 and imaging often done though not required in Table 4.3.

**Table 4.2: Common clinical indications for imaging.**

**(CT/MR) of brain**
- Stroke, head injury, dementia, late onset seizures, partial seizures
- Wherever a focal neurological deficit is detected (monoparesis, papilledema)
- Progressive headache with added features like vomiting, blurring of vision suggestive of raised intracranial pressure.
- MR Spine
  - Spinal cord disorders—demyelination, tumors
  - Symptomatic lumbar disc prolapse

**Table 4.3: Usually not recommended but often done!**

**MR brain**
- Isolated giddiness, syncope
- Migraine, tension headache
- Parkinson's disease and other movement disorders (like tremors, chorea, athetosis)
- Vague intermittent tingling, numbness occurring in different parts of the body
- Absence epilepsy, juvenile myoclonic epilepsy.

**MR spine**
- Backache, neck pain with no neurologic symptoms or signs.

*Case History*: A 58-year-old male-diabetic of ten years duration-presented with back pain and leg pain and difficulty in walking of three months duration. MR lumbar spine was done, which showed L4-5 disc prolapse and was advised surgery. Examination showed that the difficulty in walking was due to sensory ataxia because of diabetic sensory neuropathy. The backache and leg pain were not responsible for difficulty in walking.

It is important to understand what the problem is and what this is due to rather than depend on the investigative findings.

## Electroencephalogram (EEG)

Electroencephalogram records the normal and abnormal electrical activity of the brain (encephalon) (Fig. 4.6).

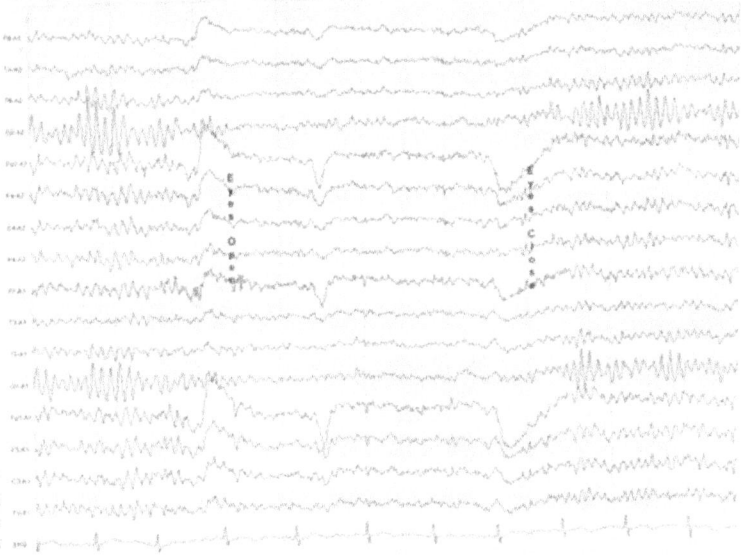

Fig. 4.6: EEG—normal.

Indications for EEG (Table 4.4) and EEG when not required (Table 4.5) are given below:

### Table 4.4: Common indications for EEG.

- After a clinical diagnosis of epilepsy, to find out the type of epilepsy (absences, JME, CPS — all have distinctive EEG changes)
- Suspected organic brain syndrome (e.g. altered behavior, memory disturbances, fluctuating conscious levels)
- In ICU where a patient is unconscious with no specific diagnosis, EEG monitoring is done to diagnose nonconvulsive status epilepticus.

## Investigations

**Table 4.5: EEG usually not recommended but often done.**
- Transient loss of consciousness
- Giddiness
- Headache
- All types of jerky movements (here it should be emphasized that epilepsy is a clinical diagnosis and EEG is only supportive and by itself is not diagnostic).

**Electroneuromyography (ENMG)** has two components EMG (electromyography), which consists of the study of the muscle by needle technique. EMG identifies primary muscle disease (myopathy, polymyositis). Nerve conduction, studies the function of the nerves—sensory and motor and when affected "neuropathy" can differentiate between axonal involvement (axonopathy) and myelin disorders (demyelinating neuropathy). What is important is the clinical application of the nerve conduction studies. They may be abnormal in elderly and in diabetic patients with no clinical correlates and they may be normal in clinically apparent neuropathies because a few large myelinated fibers are sufficient to give normal velocities. One should be aware of these limitations or else a wrong diagnosis will be made, based simply on investigations!

Indications for NCV and when not required are given in Tables 4.6 and 4.7 respectively.

**Table 4.6: Indications for NCV (nerve conduction velocity).**
- Wherever a clinical diagnosis of neuropathy (sensory/motor) is suspected
- Radiculopathy—Guillain-Barre (GB) syndrome.

**Table 4.7: NCV often asked but not required.**
- Any patient with "jum-jum" sensation in the hands or feet
- Intermittent numbness of one half of the body or one complete limb (clinically not peripheral neuropathy).

Indications for EMG are shown in Table 4.8.

**Table 4.8: Indications for EMG.**
- Clinical diagnosis of myopathy—muscle disease is suspected, e.g. polymyositis, muscular dystrophy
- Repetitive nerve stimulation test is an extremely important tool to diagnose myasthenia.

### HOW TO REFER FOR ENMG?

As with all investigations a brief history and provisional diagnosis—neuropathy, myopathy—is required to know whether only nerve conduction velocity (NCV) is enough or EMG to be done. Often times a patient with muscle disease is referred for NCV, which may be normal. Unless specifically asked EMG is not done.

In case of radiculopathy (GB syndrome) F&H responses have to be done, not just nerve conduction alone.

## CAROTID DOPPLER STUDY

This is an over-used and much abused investigation. Anyone with giddiness/syncope or any "cerebral event": particularly after the age of 50 years is referred for this study. It is but natural that the lumen of blood vessels narrow as one grows old. You cannot expect any blood vessel in the body to be as clean and patent at the age of 60 years, as it was at the age of 20 years! The brain has an excellent system of collateral circulation in the form of circle of Willis, so much so that occlusion of one vessel may be totally asymptomatic. Mere narrowing of the vessel or even occlusion of the vessel does not necessarily imply that the patient's symptoms are related to that.

Tables 4.9 and 4.10 give the indications for Carotid Doppler study and when not required respectively.

**Table 4.9: Indications for carotid Doppler study.**
- TIA in carotid system
- Ischemic stroke with good functional recovery
- In both instances, Doppler study is to identify significant stenotic lesions so that carotid intervention can be planned to prevent the *next stroke*.

**Table 4.10: Carotid Doppler studies—usually not recommended but often done!**
- Giddiness
- Transient loss of consciousness
- Memory impairment
- Completed and *enduring disabling* ischemic stroke
- Cerebral hemorrhagic stroke
- Vertebrobasilar territory stroke.

## ANTIEPILEPTIC DRUG (AED) ASSAY

This is an another investigation that is overused and abused. Some clinicians while treating patients with epilepsy, routinely ask for antiepileptic drug levels and worse still, adjust the drug dosage on the basis of the drug level! If a patient's seizures are well controlled, no matter what the drug level is, there is no need to tamper with the dosage. Similarly if the patient has no clinical side effects there is no need to reduce the dosage even if the drug levels are beyond the therapeutic range. Then one might ask, what is the utility of this test; well, it has a specific and limited value. For example, if a patient has disabling side effects and is on more than one antiepileptic drug, in order to know which drug is causing the side effects, AED assay is useful. The other situation is to know the compliance; when seizures are not well controlled in spite of medication then the drug level will suggest whether the patient has been taking the medicines regularly or not. Routine use of antiepileptic drug assay is totally unwarranted.

**Cerebrospinal Fluid (CSF):** For a non-neurologist and the patient alike, a lumbar puncture is a "major" procedure fraught with danger. CSF examination is the *gold standard* investigation for diagnosis of meningitis and encephalitis. In the olden days the CSF would be kept for observation and 24 hours later if a "cobweb" formation is seen, the diagnosis was tuberculous (TB) meningitis! It is heartening to note that today we have a range of investigations that can be done on CSF which can suggest a specific causative diagnosis.

The CSF may show "nonspecific" changes very similar to the ECG showing nonspecific ST-T changes, such as a slight rise in protein (less than 100 mg), a slight rise in cell count (20-40) with normal sugar values does not mean any specific diagnosis. Often these nonspecific changes are misinterpreted as evidence of TB meningitis. For more details on CSF analysis, see Chapter 23.

Indications for Lumbar puncture (Table 4.11), important points (Table 4.12) and clinical features of post LP headache (Table 4.13) are given below:

**Table 4.11: Lumbar puncture—CSF analysis indications.**
- Neuro infection (viral, bacterial, fungal)
- Subarachnoid hemorrhage
- Carcinomatous meningitis
- Demyelinating disorder—(MS—oligoclonal bands)
- GB syndrome (CIDP—for albuminocytological dissociation)

**Table 4.12: CSF examination—points to note.**
- CSF examination is mandatory and is the gold standard investigation for diagnosis of meningitis and encephalitis
- Nonspecific CSF changes, like nonspecific ST-T changes in ECG, are common which require clinical correlation/a repeat CSF examination
- Presence of antibodies in CSF does not necessarily give the final diagnosis
- Repeated CSF examination required for the diagnosis of carcinomatous meningitis.

**Table 4.13: Clinical features of post LP headache.**
- Dull occipito-frontal headache
- Starts within 48 hours after LP
- Characteristically headache starts in sitting/standing posture
- Disappears in lying down posture
- Neck stiffness may be present
- Spontaneous recovery within a week
- Symptomatic management with analgesics and bed rest
- Rarely epidural blood patch.

Post lumbar puncture (LP) headache occurs in 10-20%.
Table 4.14 shows various incidental findings.

**Table 4.14: Incidental findings in investigation – Relevant only if the clinical diagnosis is corroborative.**

- **MR brain**
  - Calcified granuloma
  - Lacunar infarcts
  - White matter hyper intensities
  - Cortical atrophy
  - Small benign tumors e.g. meningioma, neurofibroma
- **MR spine**
  - Cervical: C 5–6; C 6–7—Disc prolapse even causing indentations of cervical cord,
    Myelomalacia, cervical canal stenosis
  - Lumbar: L4–5, L5–S1, disk prolapse
    Sequestration of disc in lumbar canal
    Lumbar canal stenosis
- Nerve conduction studies
  - Carpal Tunnel syndrome (delayed conduction at wrist)
  - Peripheral neuropathy
- EEG
  - Nonspecific sharp waves, slow waves
  - Occasional spike wave discharges
- **Carotid/vertebral Doppler study**
  - Narrowing of blood vessels—carotid, vertebral arteries
  - Hypoplastic vertebral artery

# CHAPTER 5

# Headache

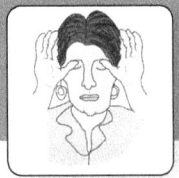

*Doctor I have a severe headache.*
*Doctor I have been having this headache for several years, please do something about it.*

Migraine is a very common diagnosis offered for a variety of headaches!

Headache is a very common complaint, though many people do not see a doctor but manage it themselves with over the counter (OTC) analgesics or even a strong cup of coffee. This is because the commonest cause of headache is what is called "muscle tension headache"/"tension type headache" which comes episodically and is self-limiting.

The usual route taken by a person with recurrent/chronic headache is self-medication → family physician → ophthalmologist → ENT surgeon → physician → orthopedic surgeon, and finally a neurologist. In the process of going through these steps there would be a variety of diagnosis, unnecessary and expensive investigations including CT, MRI and prescription of spectacles, correction of deviated nasal septum, low BP/high BP diagnosis, cervical spondylosis, etc.

## ORIGIN OF HEADACHE

The pain sensitive extracranial structures are periosteum of skull, muscles of the cranium (temporalis frontalis and occipitalis muscles) and extracranial blood vessels (temporal arteries). The intracranial pain sensitive structures are meninges, dural sinuses blood vessels, and sensory nerves (Vth cranial nerve).

The first step in the analysis of headache is to find out whether its origin is intracranial or extracranial. The adage "Tell me who your friends are and I will tell you who you are", holds good in clinical neurology. If the headache is accompanied by symptoms of intracranial localization like diplopia, blurring of vision, seizures, hemiparesis, ataxia, cranial nerve palsy etc. or signs of raised intracranial pressure like papilledema, it is of intracranial localization (Table 5.1).

### Table 5.1: Headache localization.

| Intracranial | Extracranial |
|---|---|
| ❏ Holocranial, frontal, occipital | ❏ Holocranial or temporal, frontal, vertex |
| ❏ Progressive in duration and intensity | ❏ Unilateral |
| ❏ Associated vomiting +/− | ❏ Episodic, varying in intensity |
|  | ❏ Associated vomiting +/− |
| ❏ Neurological features<br>  ▪ Seizures<br>  ▪ Altered sensorium<br>  ▪ Hemiparesis<br>  ▪ Cranial nerve palsies | Nil |

The useful clinical rule is that longer the duration of headache lesser is the possibility of intracranial pathology, in other words careful history and good neurological examination will differentiate between intra and extracranial headache and imaging of the head is often unnecessary (Table 5.1).

A patient consults a doctor in the following situations:
When the headache is
❏ Sudden and severe
❏ Recurrent and frequent
❏ Chronic and prolonged.

## NEW ONSET SUDDEN SEVERE HEADACHE

How do we approach this patient?

The first thing is to rule out major disorders like subarachnoid hemorrhage and acute pyogenic meningitis (Table 5.2).

### Table 5.2: When should CT/MRI scan be asked for a patient with headache?

❏ Headache associated with neurological symptoms or signs (diplopia, dysarthria, ataxia, papilledema, loss of consciousness, etc.)
❏ Change in the pattern of headache, e.g. patient may have ten years history of tension headache but of late it has become more severe, more prolonged and has a different quality altogether
❏ Progressively worsening headache
❏ New onset severe headache
❏ Headache associated with fever, vomiting, etc.

Subarachnoid hemorrhage should be suspected when there is an *abrupt onset of severe headache with vomiting and neck stiffness*. If the patient is sick with fever, acute pyogenic meningitis should be considered. Imaging of brain particularly CT head scan would be helpful to detect subarachnoid blood. A lumbar puncture will confirm the presence of pyogenic meningitis. If the imaging of brain and cerebrospinal fluid (CSF) is normal then one can relax as ominous conditions are ruled out; now consider primary headaches.

*Case History:* 35-year-old-female presented with abrupt onset of seizure, headache and vomiting followed an hour later by confusion and disorientation.

Examination showed neck stiffness, was afebrile; plain CT head scan revealed subarachnoid blood (Fig. 5.1).

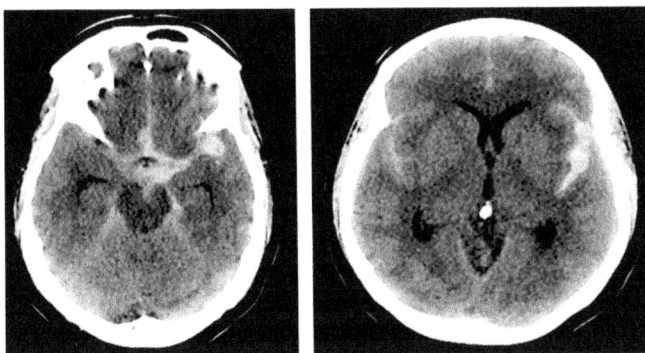

**Fig. 5.1:** CT head scan—subarachnoid hemorrhage.

*Diagnosis:* Primary subarachnoid hemorrhage.

*Case History:* A 22-year-old male engineering student presented with episodic generalized headache of four weeks duration. The headaches were moderately severe. He used to take analgesics so that he could attend classes. At this point of time, from the history, the headache appeared to be extra--cranial, probably tension headache. He was prescribed amitriptyline. CT head scan was normal. A week later the headaches became more progressive and intense along with vomiting. With the appearance of vomiting the scene changed and it was thought to be extracranial headache of migraine type (tension headaches do not produce vomiting) or due to an intracranial cause. As the CT head scan done recently was normal he continued symptomatic therapy. Two weeks later on a background of persistent headache and occasional vomiting he developed diplopia. This symptom confirms that there is an intracranial disease which is responsible for the slow progression of headache, vomiting and double vision (examination showed right 6th nerve palsy). Whenever a new symptom develops, it is mandatory to repeat the imaging and this time an MRI brain was done which too was normal! The next important investigation when an imaging is normal with a definite intracranial disease is CSF analysis—which too was well within normal limits. At this stage he was reexamined and in addition to 6th nerve palsy he had developed bilateral early papilledema, suggestive of raised intracranial pressure which prompted the possibility of cerebral venous thrombosis and hence MRI scan was repeated with MRI venogram. Lo and behold it showed thrombosis of sagittal and transverse sinus confirming the diagnosis (Fig. 5.2).

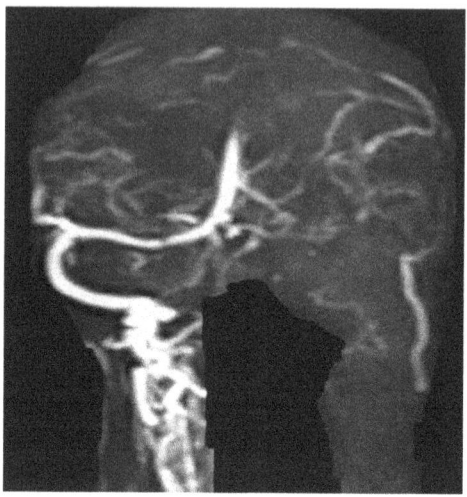

**Fig. 5.2:** MR venography: Thrombosis of superior sagittal sinus, left transverse and sigmoid sinuses.

***Diagnosis:*** Cerebral venous thrombosis.

**Message:** As new symptoms develop, one should revise the diagnosis, and reinvestigate.

The headaches are classified into Primary or Secondary type (Table 5.3).

| Table 5.3: Classification of headache. | |
|---|---|
| *Primary* | *Secondary* |
| (No neurological deficit) | (Neurological symptoms/signs) |
| a. Tension type headache | |
| b. Migraine | ❑ Subarachnoid haemorrhage |
| c. Cluster headache | ❑ Meningitis – acute/chronic |
| d. Indomethacin responsive headache | ❑ Intracranial space occupying lesion (tumor, subdural hematoma) |
| e. Chronic daily headache | |

### Tension Type Headache (TTH)

This is the commonest type of headache encountered in clinical practice. The symptoms are classified as i. episodic tension headache when the headache lasts for a few days and ii. recurs and chronic tension type headache when the headache lasts for more than 15 days in a month (Table 5.4).

### Table 5.4: Clinical features of tension type headache.

- Tight band-like sensation over the head as though somebody is pressing hard
- Bilateral distribution
- Many patients have localization of the headache to the vertex
- Fluctuating headache—becoming more severe by evening
- Generally not disabling, which means patient is able to carry on all daily activities in spite of "severe headache"
- Most important distinguishing features from migraine are that there are no associated features like nausea, vomiting, phonophobia, photophobia.
- Other associated features like chest pain, acidity, back pain, etc. are usually present.

I usually explain to the patient that stress is responsible for the release of some chemicals in the brain which in turn act on various organs in the body giving rise to a host of clinical symptoms which are genuinely felt by the patient. Generally the response of the patient is that they do not have any "tension". I then explain to them that tension does not mean major issues like loss of large amount of money or bereavement but it can also be day to day problems like maid not turning up, children not returning from school on time, etc. which cause stress in individuals who are prone for it. In Type A personality one is anxious, tense and on the edge all the time whereas a person with Type B personality is easy going, relaxed and not unduly concerned about the outcome; therefore it can be said that tension headache depends on the personality of the individual. It is the individual who interprets an event as tension.

**Management:** An acute episode is managed with acetaminophen, paracetamol, nonsteroidal anti-inflammatory drugs (NSAIDs).

**Prophylactic therapy** consists of Amitriptyline, Duloxetine, relaxation therapy, yoga, meditation (Table 5.5).

## Migraine

There are two types of migraine.

### Migraine without Aura

- Unilateral throbbing
- Moderate to severe pain
- Nausea—Vomiting
- Photophobia, phonophobia
- Aggravated by physical activity.

### Migraine with Aura

- Transient visual, speech, sensory symptoms
- Headache as described above, follows

**Management of Acute Attack** is by analgesics like acetaminophen, paracetamol, NSAIDS.

If no response to the above, ergot preparation, 1–2 mg orally or triptans.

To abort severe attack, intranasal sumatriptan spray 5–20 mg or subcutaneous injection sumatriptan 6 mg, Rizatriptan 10 mg sublingual.

In addition antiemetics, e.g. metoclopramide 5–10 mg or prochlorperazine 10–25 mg.

**Prophylactic therapy** to be considered when a person has 3 or more migraine headaches per month for three consecutive months. There is no point in starting prophylactic therapy if someone has one or two headaches once in two months and hence it is important to maintain a diary of headaches. *The duration of treatment is for a minimum of 3-4 months of headache free period* (Table 5.5).

**Table 5.5: Prophylactic therapy for migraine.**
- Propranolol 40–120 mg per day
- Topiramate 25–100 mg hs
- Valproate 200–400 mg bd
- Flunarizine 5–15 mg hs
- Amitriptyline 10–50 mg hs

If one drug fails the other can be tried. The choice of drug also depends on the comorbid features, e.g. if the person has migraine + epilepsy, use valproate, for migraine + obesity use topiramate, for migraine + essential tremor use propranolol.

It is better to avoid propranolol in patients who have asthma and valproate in obese individuals.

Infrequently migraine may be confused with occipital seizures.

The differentiating features between migraine and occipital seizures are as follows. The treatment is entirely different hence correct diagnosis is mandatory (Table 5.6).

**Table 5.6: Differentiating features of migraine and occipital seizures.**

|  | Migraine | Occipital seizures |
|---|---|---|
| Visual symptoms | Black and white | Multicolored |
|  | Flashes, linear zigzag | Circular |
|  | Begins at center and spreads peripherally | Begins laterally |
|  | Scotoma common | Uncommon |
| Frequency | Infrequent | Frequent |
| On set | Gradual | Abrupt |
| Duration | Prolonged: 15–60 minutes | Brief 30–120 seconds |

**Basilar Migraine:** Basilar migraine has features like severe unilateral occipital headache and features of basilar artery insufficiency, e.g. bilateral visual blurring at times leading to total blindness and associated brain stem symptoms with altered sensorium.

Differentiating features of tension type headache and migraine are mentioned in Table 5.7.

**Table 5.7: Differentiating features—tension type headache and migraine.**

| | Tension type headache | Migraine |
|---|---|---|
| Character | Band like around head over vertex Tightening sensation F > M | Unilateral throbbing |
| Gender | | F > M |
| Duration | Several hours to days | 1–2 hours |
| Periodicity | Frequent | Infrequent |
| Associated symptoms | Giddiness Acidity Palpitation Not aggravated by routine activities | Nausea, vomiting Photophobia Phonophobia Prefers to be left alone |
| Treatment | Tricyclic Antidepressants | Ergot preparations Triptans |

*Cluster Headache*

Cluster headache—as the name implies headaches occur frequently in a cluster (Table 5.8).

**Table 5.8: Clinical features of cluster headache.**

- M > F
- Unilateral, severe, retro-orbital.
- Often in the night
- Patient restless pacing up and down (note, in migraine patient prefers complete rest)
- Occurs in a cluster of two to six times per night repeating every night over the next 4–6 weeks
- Photophobia, phonophobia, when it occurs is unilateral (note in migraine it is bilateral)
- Autonomic features—lacrimation, nasal congestion, conjunctival injection

**Management**
- **Acute attack**—100% oxygen inhalation 10-12 liters per minute for 15 to 20 minutes.
  Sumatriptan subcutaneous 6 mg or nasal spray 20 mg.
- **Prophylactic**—as cluster headache continues for several weeks the following are used.
  Prednisolone 60-80 mg daily; taper off over two to three weeks.
  Verapamil/lithium along with steroid; taper over six weeks.

### Indomethacin Responsive Paroxysmal Hemicrania

This is a unique type of headache, quite severe, does not respond to analgesics, ergot or tranquilizers. The patient is usually made to undergo several investigations including lumbar puncture (LP) CSF because of the severity, *responds dramatically to Indomethacin and hence the name* (Table 5.9).

**Table 5.9: Clinical features of paroxysmal hemicrania.**
- F > M
- Unilateral, retro-orbital, occurring in paroxysms of 5 to 15 minutes, 10–15/day
- Severe
- With autonomic features.

**Management**

As the name implies excellent response only to indomethacine 25-75 mg tds; taper over four to eight weeks and maintain at minimum possible dose.

Cluster headaches and paroxysmal hemicrania have to be differentiated (Table 5.10) as the management is totally different.

**Table 5.10: Differential features of cluster headache and paroxysmal hemicrania.**

|  | Cluster headache | Paroxysmal hemicrania (indomethacin responsive) |
|---|---|---|
| Gender | M > F | F > M |
| Type of pain | Stabbing, boring | Throbbing, boring, stabbing |
| Severity | Moderate to severe | Moderate to severe |
| Site | Orbit, temple | Orbit, temple |
| Attack frequency | 2–3/night and day | 5–40 |
| Duration of attack | 10–30 min | 2–10 min |
| Autonomic features | Present | Present |
| Indomethacin response | – | Good |
| Prophylactic treatment | Verapamil Lithium | Indomethacin |

### Chronic Daily Headache

Chronic daily headache lasting for 15 days or more/month is a combination of chronic migraine and chronic tension headache. Management consists of using the same medicines used for prophylactic migraine/tension headache, e.g. amitriptyline, flunarizine, valproate, topiramate.

# Headache

***Case History:*** A 35-year-old female complained of chronic headache of ten years duration which was initially episodic; now chronic for the previous six months. The headache is holocranial, fluctuating in intensity, more so in the evenings, with varying locations—sometimes over the vertex and at other times in the frontal or occipital area. When asked about the intensity she says "quite severe all through"; the headache is severe even when I am talking to her! though to me she looks very comfortable. When asked "how often do you have to retire to bed leaving your work" she replies that she can continue with her activities and has never taken leave from office or rested at home because of her many responsibilities. Further enquiry revealed that she also suffers from "gastric" problem. This is a typical scenario of chronic tension type headache, best addressed by amitriptyline, counseling, and yoga.

***Message:*** Chronic headache not affecting the daily activities and associated with other stress symptoms like gastric problem is suggestive of tension type headache.

**Table 5.11: Trigeminal neuralgia: Clinical features.**

- Unilateral sudden onset
- Trigeminal nerve usually 2nd or 3rd division
- Electric shock-like pain
- Lasts for several seconds
- Triggered by washing face, brushing, eating, swallowing water, breeze, shaving
- No neurologic deficit
- Trigeminal sensory—Normal
- Spontaneous remission—only to recur later
- ***Cause:*** In few patients vascular compression of trigeminal nerve at root entry zone
- Others—not known

## Management of Trigeminal Neuralgia

- Pharmacotherapy—Carbamazepine, Phenytoin, Gabapentin, Baclofen
  The dose to be titrated till pain free and continued for one month pain free period and gradually tapered by one tablet every month. If pain recurs, go back to previous dose
- Radio frequency lesion of affected division of trigeminal nerve → relief from pain for several months
- Percutaneous balloon compression
- Surgical treatment—Microvascular decompression.

Temporal arteritis is an inflammatory disease of the temporal artery.
Trigeminal neuralgia and temporal arteritis have distinct clinical manifestations and management (Tables 5.11 and 5.12).

**Table 5.12: Clinical features of Temporal arteritis (Giant Cell Arteritis).**

- Age above 50 years
- Unilateral temporal headache, non-throbbing, dull, increases at night
- Tender temporal artery
- Associated features—polymyalgia rheumatica, fever, weight loss
- Increased ESR above 50 millimeters at the end of one hour
- Dramatic response to steroids. Start with 60–80 mg Prednisolone and taper over 4–6 weeks
- 50% of the patients develop blindness due to ophthalmic artery involvement; need to continue small dose of steroids

# CHAPTER 6

# Dizziness / Vertigo

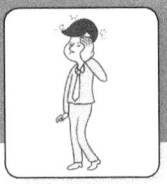

*Dr I feel giddy/vertigo/dizzy*

Giddiness is one of the common symptoms encountered in neurological practice. Patients use different terms like giddiness, dizziness, floating sensation, imbalance, light headedness, darkening in front of eyes, etc. The first thing one should do is to differentiate a ***true vertigo*** from the rest of the crowd.

The approach to the problem is to determine whether it is (Table 6.1):
- True vertigo
- Presyncope
- Imbalance (ataxia)
- Psychogenic.

Table 6.1: Differential features of vertigo, presyncope, ataxia, psychogenic causes.

| *I. True vertigo* (Vestibular system) | *II. Presyncope* (Cerebral hypoxemia) | *III. Ataxia* | *IV. Psychogenic* |
|---|---|---|---|
| *Symptoms* <br> ❏ Any posture <br> ❏ True vertigo (Spinning) <br> ❏ Vomiting <br> ❏ Sweating | *Symptoms* <br> ❏ Usually on change of posture/standing <br> ❏ Blurring of vision <br> ❏ Dizziness <br> ❏ Sinking feeling | *Symptoms* <br> ❏ Only on standing/ walking <br> ❏ Gait imbalance (when mild interpreted as dizziness) | *Symptoms* <br> ❏ Dizzy *all the time* <br> *Subjective Feeling of unsteadiness* |
| *Causes* <br> a. Vestibular nucleus (VBI) (brain stem symptoms and signs) <br> b. Vestibular nerve (vestibular neuritis) <br> c. Inner ear (labyrinthitis) (vertigo + hearing impairment) | *Causes* <br> a. Vasovagal <br> b. Cardiogenic <br> c. Postural hypotension <br> d. Carotid hypersensitivity | *Causes* <br> a. Vestibular <br> b. Sensory <br> c. Cerebellar | *Causes* <br> Anxiety <br> Hyperventilation |

## TRUE VERTIGO

True vertigo consists of *definite sense of rotation* (spinning) either of the individual or surroundings, often associated with vomiting, sweating and imbalance and is a manifestation of vestibular dysfunction.

During the period of true vertigo, a person will be unable to walk or stand without support. This means that if a patient says he has "spinning sensation" but yet is able to climb into a moving bus, it is not true vertigo! The diagnosis of true vertigo is further confirmed by associated features like nausea, vomiting and sweating.

True vertigo means the lesion is in the vestibular system—nucleus, nerve or end organ.

Further localization depends on the adage "Tell me who your friend is and I will tell you who you are" (Table 6.2).

| Table 6.2: Localization for true vertigo. | |
|---|---|
| **Structure involved** | **Clinical features** |
| a. Vestibular nucleus in the brain stem | Associated brain stem symptoms like diplopia, dysarthria, hemiparesis |
| b. Vestibular nerve in its course | Pure vertigo |
| c. Labyrinth (end organ) | Associated auditory symptoms—hearing impairment, fullness of ear |

The vestibular system involvement is characterized by the presence of nystagmus.

*Nystagmus* has two components—quick jerky movement and a slow correction. The direction of nystagmus is defined by the direction of quick phase.

a. **Spontaneous:** When nystagmus is elicited on looking straight it is suggestive of a vestibular dysfunction.

*Central*: The nystagmus quality is purely vertical or torsional, not affected by visual fixation.

*Peripheral*: Nystagmus is unidirectional, horizontal or torsional, increased in the direction of fast phase. Peripheral nystagmus is reduced by visual fixation, e.g. while doing an optic fundus examination by closing the other eye.

b. **Gaze evoked nystagmus** is almost always central or drug induced, changes direction with direction of gaze; is due to brain stem, cerebellar disorders or toxic metabolic conditions. If it is symmetric, it is due to toxic metabolic causes and if asymmetric it is due to an unilateral lesion of brain stem or cerebellum (Table 6.3).

### Table 6.3: Clinical features of central versus peripheral nystagmus.

| | Peripheral | Central |
|---|---|---|
| Latency (time to onset of nystagmus/vertigo) | 5–30 seconds | No latency |
| Symptoms | Intense vertigo, vomiting, short lived | Less intense, constant infrequent vomiting |
| Direction | Unidirectional, fast component towards the normal ear | Gaze evoked, changes direction |
| Type | Horizontal with a torsional component, never vertical | Can be in any direction—horizontal or vertical |
| Duration | 20–40 seconds | Persists |
| Effect of visual fixation | Suppressed | Not suppressed |
| Fatigability | Yes | No |
| Auditory symptoms Deafness or tinnitus | May be present | Absent |
| Other neurologic features | Absent | Often present—UMN, cerebellar features, diplopia |
| Common causes | BPPV, Ménière's disease | Vertebrobasilar insufficiency (VBI), demyelination in brain stem (MS) |

Common causes of vertigo are mentioned in Table 6.4.

### Table 6.4: Common causes of true vertigo.

**Peripheral causes**
Benign paroxysmal positional vertigo (BPPV)
Vestibular neuritis
Labyrinthitis
Ménière's disease
Acoustic neuroma
Aminoglycoside toxicity
Otitis media

**Central causes**
Migrainous vertigo
Brain stem ischemia, demyelination

***Benign paroxysmal positional vertigo (BPPV)*** is the commonest disorder seen in day-to-day practice.

Typically the symptoms are abrupt onset of incapacitating true vertigo occurring while the patient is turning and getting out of the bed (while waking up in the morning). The patient goes back to bed and is scared, thinking that he is having a stroke. Characteristically the vertigo lasts for few seconds. After a few minutes when he tries to get up the vertigo recurs. After resting for some time, he gets out of the bed and is relieved to note that he is ok. However when he bends his head to wash his face at the washbasin the vertigo recurs again. The vertigo is brought about by *change in position of the head* like turning in the bed, bending forwards to brush the teeth or bending to tie shoe laces or pick up an object from the floor, the vertigo lasts only for a few seconds. The natural history is spontaneous recovery over the next four to six days.

The diagnosis can be confirmed by asking the patient to lie down and turn to either side and when the patient complains of vertigo observe for horizontal or rotary nystagmus. The episode can also be observed by Dix-Hallpike maneuver, wherein the patient is asked to sit on the bed with his head turned to 45° and the examiner holds the head and gently brings it down supine with the head hanging below the bed, which elicits vertigo and nystagmus.

Mechanism for this condition is floating of calcium carbonate crystals (otoconia) in semicircular canals which are displaced from utricle and saccule. So the treatment consists of repositioning of these crystals by Epley maneuver followed at home by Brandt-Daroff exercises (Fig. 6.1).

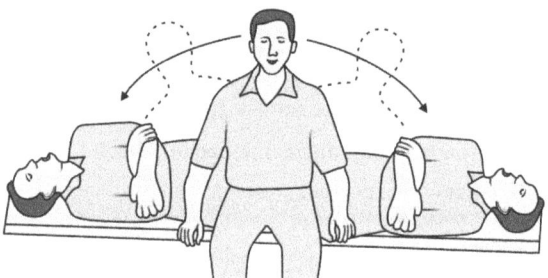

**Fig. 6.1:** Brandt-Daroff exercises.

Sit upright on the bed, lie down to one side keeping the head at 45°, wait till giddiness disappears, count slowly till seven; come back to upright position, count till seven slowly; lie down on the other side wait till giddiness disappears or count slowly till seven and finally back to upright position. Do this ten times each on either side and three sets per day for two weeks and once set per day for another two weeks.

Additional treatment consists of asking the patient to turn in the bed *very slowly*, sit up *gradually* and stand for *a few seconds* before walking. Vertigo suppressant drugs (cinnarizine) may be used for a short period of 7-10 days; Anxiolytics like clonazepam 0.25 mg helps alleviate the fear of vertiginous feeling.

## How to Differentiate BPPV from VBI (Vertebrobasilar Insufficiency)

Often an elderly person with BPPV is worried whether it is a stroke; in case of a stroke involving brain stem, there will be additional neurological features like diplopia, dysarthria, ataxia, hemiparesis (always remember the adage – "tell me who your friends are and I will tell who you are"). When vertigo is a *stand-alone symptom*, of brief duration and related to change of position of head the diagnosis is assured and there is no need for MRI brain, MR angiography, carotid Doppler, etc. which unfortunately is often done. There are several causes of acute vertigo (Table 6.5) and vestibular neuronitis is one of them (Table 6.6).

**Table 6.5: Acute vertigo: Differential diagnosis.**

| Clinical features | | Duration | Examination |
|---|---|---|---|
| BPPV | ❑ Starts while getting out of bed<br>❑ Occurs whenever position of head is changed, e.g. bending forward, turning in bed | Few seconds to a minute | Peripheral nystagmus when the patient experiences vertigo |
| Acute vestibular neuronitis | ❑ Starts anytime<br>❑ Enduring, irrespective of position<br>❑ Ataxia, vomiting prominent | Resolves over 24–72 hours | Peripheral nystagmus |
| Acute labyrinthitis | ❑ Same as above plus hearing impairment | As above | Peripheral nystagmus |
| Brain stem ischemia (VBI) | ❑ Vertigo, vomiting, ataxia, dysarthria, dysphagia | ❑ Transient if it is TIA<br>❑ Enduring if infarct | Brain stem features—Diplopia, central nystagus dysarthria, dysphagia, ataxia, hemiparesis |

**Table 6.6: Clinical features of acute vestibular neuronitis/acute labyrinthitis.**
- Acute onset of vertigo with associated symptoms of vomiting, sweating
- Episode lasting *for few days*, disabling the person who is almost confined to bed
- If vertigo is the only symptom it is vestibular neuronitis
- If there is associated fullness of ear, hearing impairment it is Labyrinthitis.

This condition is something like Bell's palsy—a monophasic illness with spontaneous recovery. For rapid recovery a short course of steroid, prednisolone 40-60 mg/day for 8-10 days, in addition to vestibular suppressant medication is prescribed.

**Ménière's disease** is a less common type of peripheral vertigo (Table 6.7).

### Table 6.7: Clinical features of Ménière's disease.

- Episodic in nature
- Occurs once in two to six months; gradually the frequency increases
- Abrupt onset of true vertigo which is disabling with associated features of vomiting and sweating
- The episode lasts for a few hours after which the person is back to normal
  - The diagnosis is aided by associated auditory features like fullness of ear, tinnitus and hearing impairment. This can be confirmed by audiogram which shows low frequency hearing loss.

Management of acute episode, though self-limiting, may be helped by anti-vertigo and antiemetic drugs (Prochlorperazine, Ondansetron). The problem is to prevent subsequent episodes. Salt restriction in the diet, diuretics and prolonged treatment with betahistine may reduce the rate of recurrence. When the episodes are frequent intratympanic gentamycin injection (into middle ear) is helpful to prevent subsequent attacks.

## PRESYNCOPE

Dizziness, blurring of vision, sinking feeling are symptoms of presyncope and when extended, leads to syncope (falling to ground). Characteristically they occur when the patient is standing for a long time or in crowded area or due to stressful situations and is associated with nausea and sweating. (For discussion on presyncope, *see* Chapter 9.

## GAIT ATAXIA

If "giddiness" occurs only while walking or standing with *no feeling of spinning*, then it is gait imbalance and has to be further analyzed for vestibular, sensory, cerebellar ataxia. The focused neurological examination consists of walking normally, walking on heels, on toes, tandem walking, walking briskly with a quick about turn and finally standing with feet together eyes open and then eyes closed (Romberg's sign). If all these tests can be done without difficulty this means it is probably psychogenic. (For more discussion on gait imbalance, *see* Chapter 14).

## PSYCHOGENIC DIZZINESS

Patient complains of dizziness/giddiness *all the time* with varying intensity. It is not disabling and the person is able to carry out all activities as usual including climbing into a running bus! There are no associated symptoms like vomiting or sweating, but associated features of anxiety and depression like headache, acidity, chest pain, palpitation etc. are present.

Management consists of addressing the underlying anxiety. Often patients are prescribed vertigo suppressant medications and the *patient gets hooked to it* after using it for long periods of time. Some of them develop extrapyramidal features as a side effect!

***Case History:*** A 45-year-old female came with complaints of "giddiness" on walking in open spaces which worsens when crossing the street, of six months duration. She is able to walk normally within the house and there is no history of fall. Six months earlier she had a clear cut episode of benign positional vertigo, which resolved within a week. Neurological examination was unremarkable.

Clinical diagnosis was phobic disorder following an episode of positional vertigo. She had undergone several investigations including MRI brain, MR cervical spine, ENMG, vitamin B12 level, etc. She improved with anxiolytics (Clonazepam) and reassurance.

Some patients may need counseling too.

***Diagnosis:*** Phobic disorder—Agoraphobia

***Message:*** Investigations without clinical diagnosis have no meaning!

# CHAPTER 7

# Neck Pain

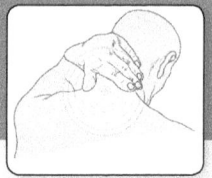

*"Doctor I have Cervical Spondylosis"*
This is a common way of presentation of today's elite patients!

First thing to realize is spondylosis itself is not a disease, it is just an age-related change, like balding of the head and greying of the hair! It causes medical problems in few individuals, even though the radiological changes can be seen invariably after the age of 50 years. These changes range from minimal spondylotic abnormalities to disc prolapse indenting the cord and even causing myelomalacia. Yet is clinically totally asymptomatic!

When a person gets up in the morning with acute pain in the neck and difficulty to move the neck it is usually due to bad posturing while sleeping. Analgesics and hot fomentation relieves the pain (Table 7.1).

**Table 7.1: Causes of neck pain.**

- Neck muscle — Sprain, injury
    - Dystonia — Idiopathic, drug induced
- Spine — Cervical spondylosis, secondaries
    - Traumatic injuries
    - Arthritis – Rheumatoid, tuberculosis, pyogenic
- Meninges — Meningitis

The common cause of *constant* neck pain *over a long period of time* is due to wrong posturing of the neck while working, especially so with today's technological advances, many people spend long hours in front of the computer, craning the neck forwards with no respite! The management consists of seat adjustments to keep the low back and the neck straight while sitting on the chair and taking some time off, about 10 minutes, every two hours during which time isometric neck exercises should be done.

**Cervical Spondylosis:** The radiological findings of cervical spondylosis is quite common after the age of 50 years. Treat the patient not the image! (Table 7.2).

**Table 7.2: Cervical spondylosis has three different manifestations.**

- Arthropathy
- Radiculopathy
- Myelopathy

1. **Spondylotic arthropathy** pain over back of head, neck, shoulder and arms, with symptoms *worsening on neck movements*. Occasionally the arthropathy pain can radiate down the upper limb. This is best managed by analgesics and once pain free, isometric neck exercises will help prevent recurrence. Cervical collar to be used *only while traveling* especially on rough roads; and is not required at other times. The collar is like a *foreign aid* and when patients get addicted to it the neck muscles will further weaken!

    **Management:** Anti-inflammatory drugs for pain relief and later isometric neck exercises.

2. **Spondylotic radiculopathy** can be due to osteophyte, disc prolapse, (usually C5-6, C6-7) pinching on the exiting nerve root. This produces severe shock like pain in the involved root, characteristically worsening on coughing, sneezing and straining. For example, if the C6 root is compressed, the radiating pain occurs from the neck downwards on the lateral side involving the thumb and index fingers, sometimes associated with persistent numbness of these two fingers. The pain appears when neck is *extended* and disappears when the neck is *flexed*. This is an important clinical test to reproduce pain.

    The radiating pain of "arthropathy" is vaguely distributed in the limb and is *not aggravated* by coughing and sneezing while the pain due to root involvement is characteristically sharp along the distribution of the root with tingling and numbness aggravated by coughing and sneezing (Table 7.3).

**Table 7.3: How to differentiate arthropathy from radiculopathy.**

| Cervical | Neck pain | Worsened by neck movement | Pain over upper limbs | Pain in the distribution of root (C6,C7) | Pain worsening by cough, sneeze |
|---|---|---|---|---|---|
| Arthropathy | + | + | + | − | − |
| Radiculopathy | + | + | + | + | + |

**Management:** For cervical radiculopathy—nerve pain killer, e.g. Gabapentin, Carbamazepine. Once the pain subsides, isometric neck exercises to prevent recurrence. Cervical collar only for travel on rough roads. Very occasionally surgery (foraminotomy) to give immediate relief from pain.

3. **Spondylotic myelopathy:** The cervical cord (corticospinal tracts, posterior column) is compressed due to disc prolapse, narrow cervical canal, ossification of posterior longitudinal ligament or a combination of all the three (Table 7.4).

### Table 7.4: Clinical features of cervical spondylotic myelopathy.
- Spastic gait
- Spastic ataxic gait
- The disability is due to spasticity
- Quadriparesis. Sensory level and bladder involvement *seldom* occur
- Surgery is indicated when the patient has disabling symptoms.

**Case History:** A 62-year-old male presented with slow progressive difficulty in walking of two years duration. Examination revealed gross spasticity of all four limbs with absent vibration and position sense in lower limbs.

*Clinical Diagnosis:*

*Step 1: Neurologic deficits:* UMN quadriparesis; with posterior column dysfunction in lower limbs.

*Step 2: Anatomical localisation:* Cervical cord.

*Step 3: Pathological diagnosis:* Chronic compression posterolaterally—spondylosis.

Investigation for anatomical localization—MRI cervical spine—showed spondylotic changes, C5-6 disc prolapse indenting the cord (Fig. 7.1).

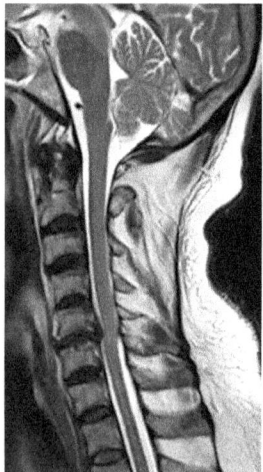
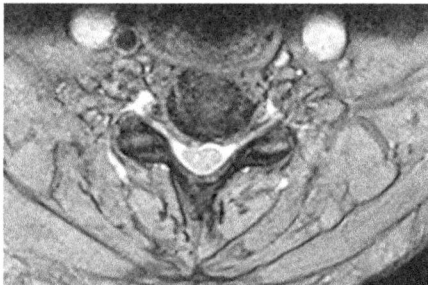

Fig. 7.1: MR cervical spine C5-6 disc prolapse indenting the cord.

As the clinical findings correlated with the imaging findings a diagnosis of cervical spondylotic myelopathy was made. He was operated upon, resulting in immense relief of symptoms.

**Diagnosis:** Cervical spondylotic myelopathy.

Magnetic resonance imaging of cervical spine is frequently done when the patient complains of giddiness. It should be emphasized that cervical

Neck Pain

spondylosis *does not produce giddiness* though this seems to be a myth perpetuated by several doctors. In the present era of over investigations, neck pain is a common symptom for which patients are over investigated with unnecessary imaging and worse still proceeding with surgery when there is no corresponding neurological dysfunction (Table 7.5).

#### Table 7.5: When to ask for MR cervical spine?
- Mere neck pain is not an indication (though done very often!)
- Myelopathy is a definite indication
- Where diagnosis of spondylosis is in doubt and other possibilities exist (e.g. TB spine, secondary deposits)
- Radiculopathy, not responding to medical treatment and contemplating surgical treatment.

Radiological diagnosis of cervical spondylosis is quite often asymptomatic. Management of cervical spondylosis depends on clinical features (Tables 7.6 to 7.9).

#### Table 7.6: Management of acute neck pain without radiculopathy.
- Symptomatic treatment with NSAID
- Spontaneous remission occurs
- Cervical collar only while traveling on rough roads (not at home or while walking)
- Cervical traction *not* recommended.

#### Table 7.7: Management of chronic neck pain without radiculopathy.
- Symptomatic treatment with NSAID
- Isometric neck exercise
- No surgery.

#### Table 7.8: Management of neck pain with radiculopathy.
- Spontaneous recovery in great majority
- Symptomatic treatment with NSAID and nerve pain killer, e.g Gabapentin, Carbamazepine
- Soft cervical collar during travel to reduce pain on neck movement
- Occasionally for immediate relief of pain—surgery.

#### Table 7.9: Indication for surgery in cervical spondylosis.
- Myelopathy
- Radiculopathy with motor weakness (e.g. C7 – Triceps)
- For immediate relief from pain in radiculopathy.

In clinical practice the two common neurological disorders which are mistakenly attributed to spondylotic changes seen on the MR scan, are motor neuron disease and Parkinson's disease.

## SPONDYLOTIC MYELOPATHY VS MOTOR NEURON DISEASE

***Case History*:** A 55-year-old male presented with progressive difficulty in walking due to stiffness of lower limb of six months duration and intermittent neck pain. In view of the spastic gait, MRI cervical spine was done, which showed spondylotic changes, with compression of cervical cord. He was operated upon but the symptoms continued to worsen.

Examination two months later showed spastic gait, *wasting of small muscles* of hand but no sensory changes.

*Step 1*: *Neurologic deficits*—Pure motor UMN in lower limb; LMN in upper limb distally

*Step 2*: *Anatomical localization*—Motor system UMN (cervical cord), LMN —D1 level

*Step 3*: *Pathological diagnosis*—Motor neuron disease.

EMG-confirmed the diagnosis as fibrillation potentials were widely distributed including in the lower limbs.

***Diagnosis*:** Motor neuron disease.

***Message*:** The common feature between MND and spondylotic myelopathy is the spastic gait. However what differentiates the two is evidence of lower motor neuron lesion in the form of wasting of small muscles of hand (C8, T1) in MND and radicular pain along C6, C7 and *posterior column sensory dysfunction* in cervical spondylotic myelopathy. MND is pure motor system disease without any sensory dysfunction (Table 7.10).

Table 7.10: Differential features of cervical spondylotic myelopathy and motor neuron disease.

|  | C. spondylotic myelopathy | Motor neuron disease |
|---|---|---|
| Spasticity lower limbs | + + | + + |
| Wasting of muscles of hand | – | + |
| Fasciculations | – | + |
| Sensory (posterior column dysfunction) in lower limbs | + | – |
| EMG | Normal | Abnormal |

## CERVICAL SPONDYLOSIS VS PARKINSON'S DISEASE

***Case History*:** A 65-year-old female presented with progressive difficulty in walking, difficulty in activities with right hand like mixing food, buttoning and pain in the neck and right shoulder. In view of stiffness of right upper and lower limbs and neck and shoulder pain, cervical spine MRI was done, which showed C5-6 disc prolapse with minimal compression of cervical cord. With a diagnosis of cervical spondylotic myelopathy, she was operated upon. Postoperative, after two weeks of rest, the symptoms worsened.

Neurological examination showed right sided rigidity (not spasticity). Diagnosis is Parkinson's disease which dramatically responded to Levodopa preparation. The diagnosis was missed as there were no tremors!

***Diagnosis*:** Parkinson's disease

***Message*:** One should differentiate spasticity from rigidity!

## CERVICAL SPONDYLOTIC RADICULOPATHY VS BRACHIAL PLEXOPATHY

***Case History*:** A 45-year-old male complained of pain over the right shoulder and upper arm, which was disturbing sleep at night. The pain had been there for 7 days followed later by difficulty in lifting the shoulder. MRI cervical spine and an MRI shoulder joint were done, both of which were non informative. Examination showed wasting of right deltoid and difficulty to abduct and flex the shoulder due to motor weakness and not because of pain. Passive movement of the shoulder was in full range, thus excluding shoulder pathology. In addition he had anesthesia of a coin size at the insertion of the deltoid.

Differential diagnosis of neck and shoulder pain are summarized in Table 7.11.

| Table 7.11: Neck and shoulder pain—differential diagnosis. | | | | |
|---|---|---|---|---|
| | *Cervical spondylosis* | *Periarthritis shoulder* | *Brachial neuritis* | *Parkinson's disease* |
| Pain | Neck and interscapular region | Shoulder pain increased on movement | Severe pain—shoulder and upper limb | Neck shoulder upper limb stiffness and pain |
| Motor weakness | Nil | Nil | Severe paralysis—shoulder, upper limb | Stiffness of upper and lower limb |
| Shoulder movements | Normal | Painful | Normal | Stiff |
| Tendon reflexes upper limb | Brisk | Normal | Biceps reduced | Normal |

*Clinical diagnosis*:
a. *Neurological deficit*: LMN paresis of abductors and flexors of right shoulder
b. *Anatomical localization*: C5, 6
c. *Pathological diagnosis*: Acute onset with severe pain—upper brachial plexopathy
d. *Etiological diagnosis*: Probably related to some viral infection and immune response.

**Diagnosis:** Right brachial plexopathy.

**Message:** Fortunately MRI cervical spine did not show C5-6 disc prolapse; otherwise he would have been operated by now! Passive movements of shoulders being complete and painless, rules out shoulder pathology which if recognized earlier would not have necessitated MRI shoulder. Severe excruciating pain over the entire right shoulder area, not limited to C7 roots is typical of brachial neuralgia and the motor weakness appreciated only when the pain spontaneously disappears.

# 8

# Back Pain

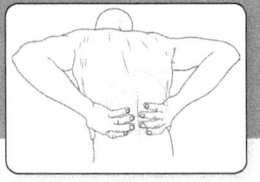

Back pain is a common symptom seen in the OPD and equally commonly mismanaged!!

The usual trend is to immediately ask for MR lumbosacral spine, and diagnose it as lumbar spondylosis. Lumbar spondylosis is not a disease but age related degenerative changes, like balding of the head and greying of hair! The radiological changes are observed almost invariably after the age of 50 years. The imaging findings may also include disk prolapse of varying degrees (in 30–40% of normal adults) and also sequestered disk floating in the lumbar canal displacing the roots without producing any clinical correlates!

## TYPES OF BACK PAIN

### Postural Back Pain

The commonest cause of back pain in the community is postural back pain/mechanical backache. Typically the pain is vague and diffuse in the lower back which increases with prolonged sitting or standing and is relieved by rest. In today's technological world a greater part of the life is spent sitting in front of a computer/TV, that too with a wrong posture which leads to back pain.

**The management** is to adjust the sitting posture in such a way that the lower back is supported by the back of the chair. Also one should not bend down while using the key board. The person should get up from the seat every two hours and take short walks, of 5 minutes, during which time they can interact with other people in office. This also increases the social interaction which is lacking in today's world! People have insulated themselves with computers, mobiles, iPads, iPhones, WhatsApp, etc. and are more informed about friends living abroad or in a different city than a person who is sitting next to him or her!! *Regular walks and back exercises are the principles of management.*

### Backache as a Part of Somatization

Although the patient starts off with complaints of back pain, from their history we get to know that they also have pain in the upper back, headache, upper limbs and so on. Such types of back pain are a part of multiple somatic symptoms due to psychological causes and respond very well to tricyclic drugs, e.g. amitriptyline. The response is seen with smaller doses, which may not be the dose for depression. The backache is vague, typically increases by evening and is experienced in all positions—sitting, standing, walking, lying down with varying severity. *The pain may fluctuate* over several days and many of them have symptoms stretching over several months to years.

### Lumbar Spondylosis

Pain in the back radiating down the lower limb can be due to arthropathy or root involvement. Then how do you differentiate between the two (Table 8.1)?

**Table 8.1: The clinical features of lumbar spondylosis.**
- Arthropathy
- Neurological involvement of a root (L5, S1)—Radiculopathy
- Multiple roots (Cauda equina syndrome)

**In arthropathy,** the pain is typically severe during the initial movement after resting and as the person becomes active, the pain disappears. Radiating pain to the lower limb is in a diffuse manner and does not worsen on coughing or sneezing. Ankle jerk is normal.

**Lumbar radiculopathy** commonly affects L5 or S1 root due to corresponding disk prolapse. The backache is accompanied by shock like or current like pain along the distribution of L5 or S1 root with tingling and numbness on the dorsum of the foot (L5) or plantar aspect (S1), and worsen on coughing or sneezing. The corresponding ankle jerk will be sluggish or absent.

When radiculopathy involves the motor root then there is neurological deficit—foot drop (weakness of dorsiflexion due to L5 root involvement) or weakness of plantar flexion (due to S1 root involvement) (Fig. 8.1 and Table 8.2).

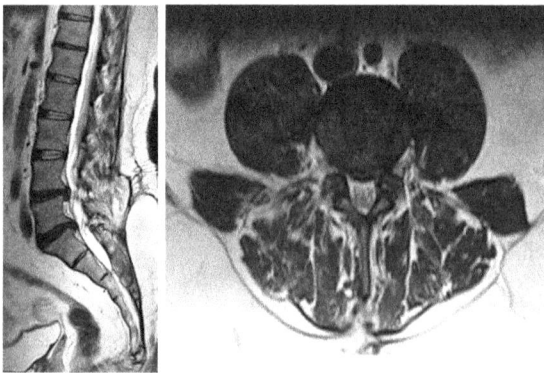

Fig. 8.1: MR lumbar spine—L4-5 disk herniation.

## Table 8.2: Differentiation between arthropathy and radiculopathy.

| Clinical features | Arthropathy | Radiculopathy |
|---|---|---|
| Pain | Maximum during initial movement after rest | Persists |
| Radiating pain | Diffuse | Shock like pain in the distribution of L5/S1 roots |
| Cough, sneeze | No change in pain | Worsens |
| Sensory, motor deficit | Absent | Present |
| Ankle jerk | Normal | Absent |

**Red flags** while in a majority of patients the back pain may be due to benign causes one should be aware of situations where it should be considered as a significant symptom. The following require attention and appropriate investigation (MR lumbosacral spine) (Table 8.3).

## Table 8.3: Red flags in back pain.

- Pain increases at night and while resting
- Worsening of pain over a short period of time (days or weeks). Mechanical, postural, psychosomatic back pain continue for a number of months or years.
- Associated neurological symptoms and signs, e.g. sensory motor deficits/bladder involvement.

### Management of Acute Low Back Pain without Neurological Deficit

The pain is typically increased by movement and reduced by rest. There is *no need* for bed rest but one should avoid position which increases pain. Early ambulation is the key, unlike in earlier days when prolonged bed rest with traction of the lower limbs was advised.

**Symptomatic management** is with NSAID, acetaminophen, and a muscle relaxant at night. Surgery is *never* indicated only for pain. Back muscle strengthening exercises should start only after the pain subsides.

*Spontaneous recovery* occurs in 3-6 weeks. There is *no need* for lumbar traction, physiotherapy, ultrasound, corset, magnet, etc.

### Management of Chronic Low Back Pain without Neurologic Deficit

Commonly seen in obese females, often with physiological disturbances, depression and chronic smoking. In such cases address these risk factors.

**The management** consists of back muscle strengthening exercises, aerobic exercises and yoga.

Symptomatic therapy for pain with NSAID like acetaminophen.

Amitriptyline is very useful in small doses of 10-25 mg/day even in the absence of clinical depression.

The role of acupuncture, massage, complementary and alternative medicine, transcutaneous electrical nerve stimulation (TENS) is unclear. Epidural steroids, facet joint injection, and trigger point injection may be useful in some patients for back pain.

There is *no role for surgery* for chronic low backache.

### Management of Acute or Chronic Low Back Pain with Radiculopathy due to Prolapsed Intervertebral Disk

*Spontaneous regression* of herniated disk occurs in 60-70% of patients over the next 3-6 months. Management consists of NSAID for immediate relief and epidural steroid, if necessary. There is no need for bed rest but only restriction of activities which aggravate pain.

The pain itself subsides without surgery over a period of time, but the patient may choose to get relief from pain much earlier by undergoing surgery.

### Management of Acute or Chronic Low Back Pain with Neurological Deficit

Motor weakness of dorsi flexor (L5) or plantar flexor (S1) is an indication for surgery. Mere absence of ankle jerk is not necessarily an indication for surgery.

**Cauda Equina Syndrome** Rarely, a massive disk prolapse into the lumbar canal can cause compression of several roots leading to LMN paralysis of both lower limbs. The syndrome consists of low back pain, asymmetric hypotonic areflexic paralysis of both lower limbs with perianal anesthesia and hypotonic bladder. For more information, refer Chapter 15.

## DOCTOR I GET PAIN IN MY LEGS WHEN I WALK

Pain in the legs on walking, relieved by rest is suggestive of ischemia to muscles (vascular cause) or ischemia of nerve roots (neurogenic).

**Lumbar canal stenosis** occurs due to narrow canal from birth which subsequently narrows further due to hypertrophied ligaments, osteophytes, disk prolapse (Fig. 8.2). Lumbar canal stenosis is *frequently asymptomatic*.

Neurogenic claudication may be a clinical manifestation.

The pain due to neurogenic claudication should be differentiated from ischemic (of muscles) claudication (Table 8.4). In both situations pain occurs in the lower limbs on walking. In neurogenic claudication the pain is due to ischemia of the lumbar roots resulting in "neuropathic" symptoms like pain, tingling, numbness and paresthesia of lower limbs which continue to worsen as the person is walking. As the sensory symptoms progress, motor symptoms of weakness of lower limbs, being unable to walk and even buckling of the knee appear. When the lumbar spine is flexed it increases the anterior posterior diameter and the pain is relieved resulting in ability to walk for a longer distance, e.g. by leaning over the pushing cart while shopping can help the person walk a longer distance than normal walking. Also pedaling a stationary bike while sitting can be done for a longer period.

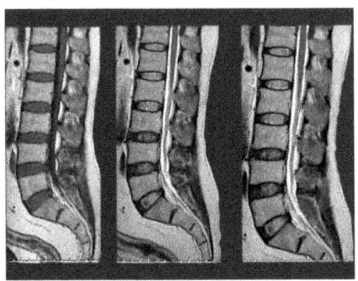
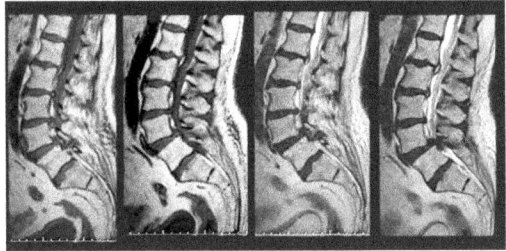

Fig. 8.2: MR lumbar spine—lumbar canal stenosis.

In vascular ischemic claudication the pain is due to ischemia of the muscles of the lower limb particularly the calf muscle and so the pain is located at the calf muscle which becomes severe as the person continues to walk.

| Table 8.4: Differential diagnosis of intermittent claudication of lower limbs. | | |
|---|---|---|
| | *Neurogenic* | *Vascular* |
| Symptoms | ❏ Tingling, numbness, paresthesia, distal later proximal<br>❏ Later on motor weakness and buckling at knee | ❏ Pain in calf muscles<br>❏ No motor weakness |
| Tendon reflexes (Knee and ankle jerk) | Sluggish/absent | Normal |
| Peripheral arteries | Normal | Feeble/absent |
| Cause | Lumbar canal stenosis | Peripheral arterial narrowing |
| Investigation | MR lumbar spine—measurement of lumbar canal | Peripheral arterial Doppler study |

# 9

# Blurring of Vision, Double Vision

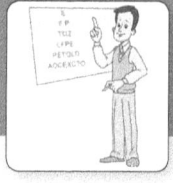

The common visual disturbances are blurring of vision, loss of vision, and double vision.

## BLURRING OF VISION

Whenever a patient complains of blurring of vision, the following tests should be done for localization (Table 9.1):
a. Check vision by closing one eye at a time. If the vision is clear with *either eye closed* and blurred with both eyes open then the diagnosis is blurring due to diplopia. There is nothing wrong with the eyes; it is due to oculomotor palsies.
b. The next step is to differentiate monocular visual disturbances from hemianopic field disturbances. If the closure of left eye shows blurring of vision in the right eye but when the right eye is closed vision is totally clear in the left eye—it means that there is a monocular visual disturbance in the right eye due to ophthalmic/neurologic causes.
c. When right side vision is affected in both eyes it means that there is right homonymous hemianopia due to a left cerebral lesion.

### Table 9.1: Visual impairment—localization.
a. Closure of either eye—Blurring disappears → III, IV, VI cranial nerve palsy
b. Uniocular visual blurring:
   i. Ophthalmic causes in retina, vitreous, lens, cornea
   ii. Neurological causes—optic nerve
c. Bilateral loss of vision:
   i. Cortical blindness, e.g. Vertebrobasilar ischemia—occipital lobe infarct
   ii. All causes of uniocular visual loss affecting both eyes
d. Hemianopia:
   i. Bitemporal—optic chiasma (pituitary tumor)
   ii. Homonymous hemianopia (contralateral cerebral hemisphere), e.g. cerebral infarct

## HOW TO ASSESS VISION?

Vision is tested in each eye, at the bed side, for distant vision and for near vision.

When unable to read, both distant and near letters, the next thing to do is to count the fingers at a distance of six feet, three feet and one foot. When this too is not feasible, hand movements at six feet, three feet and one foot should be carried out. Finally the minimum vision is assessed by perception of bright light when shone into the eye. Total loss of vision is when perception of light is absent. To test this the room *should be dark and the torch light bright!*

## TRANSIENT VISUAL DISTURBANCES

### Monocular Transient Visual Loss

- Amaurosis fugax (TIA of retina): due to emboli from carotid artery blocking central retinal artery; contralateral hemiparesis may be present
- Retinal migraine.

### Bilateral Transient Visual Loss

- TIA-VBI involving both visual cortices
- Basilar migraine
- Papilledema—raised intracranial pressure
- Hypotension, hypoperfusion.

## ENDURING MONOCULAR VISUAL LOSS

**Monocular visual disturbances** can be due to **ophthalmic causes** involving the media—cornea, anterior chamber, lens, vitreous, detachment of retina, macular diseases, **neurological causes** due to optic nerve involvement from its origin at the retina to its junction with optic chiasma (Tables 9.2 and 9.3).

**Table 9.2: Vascular causes of monocular visual disturbances.**

i. Anterior ischemic optic neuropathy (AION)
   Due to posterior ciliary artery insufficiency which supplies the optic disk
   - Age > 50 years
   - Associated—HBP, diabetes, dyslipidemia
   - Sudden painless loss of vision
   - Swollen pale optic disk with splinter hemorrhages
   - Temporal arteritis associated in 10%.
ii. Central retinal artery occlusion results in ischemic optic neuropathy with painless acute loss of vision and edematous retina with cherry red appearance of fovea.
iii. Central retinal vein occlusion, multiple hemorrhages in retina, dilated retinal veins, macular edema, cotton wool spots and central scotoma with preserved peripheral vision.

**Table 9.3: Clinical features of optic neuritis.**
- Pain behind the eye, worsened by ocular movements
- Blurring of vision/total loss of vision.
- Optic disk may look normal, if the lesion is much behind and blurred, if it is close to the disk
- The pupil will be dilated and unresponsive to light only when there is a near total loss of vision.

## Investigations

The localization to optic nerve can be confirmed by visual evoked response and MR optic nerve—plain and contrast (Fig. 9.1). The condition resolves spontaneously over a week or two. However for rapid recovery IV methyl prednisolone 1 gm daily should be given for three days followed by oral prednisolone, rapidly tapered over two weeks (Fig. 9.1).

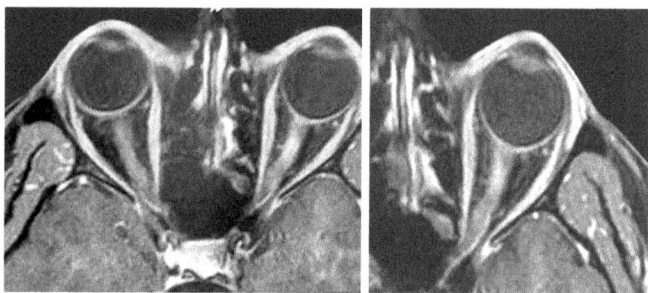

**Fig. 9.1:** MR orbits—left optic neuritis.

## Is This Isolated Optic Neuritis or Part of MS/NMO?

The answer can be got by careful enquiry about the past incidence of involvement of the eye, brainstem, or spinal cord ;then suggest an MR imaging of brain and spinal cord to look for subclinical lesions. If present, appropriate disease modifying therapy should be initiated. Clinically definite MS follows first attack of optic neuritis in 30-50% of patients.

**In optic neuropathy**, the visual loss is gradual, unlike in vascular/ inflammatory conditions mentioned above (Table 9.4).

**Table 9.4: Causes of optic neuropathy.**
- Infections:
  - Toxoplasmosis
  - Herpes
- Nutritional deficiency, B12 deficiency
- Toxins: Carbon monoxide, ethylene glycol, methanol, tobacco
- Drugs: Ethambutol, clioquinol, isoniazid, amiodarone, methotrexate
- Chemotherapeutic agents: Vincristine, cisplatin, carboplatin, paclitaxel
- Lebers hereditary optic neuropathy
  *Always look for a treatable cause*

## Visual Field Defects

**Hemianopia** is more common, in clinical practice, along with hemiplegia where visual pathways are affected in the temporoparietal region supplied by carotid system. If a patient has right hemiplegia, often, he also has right hemianopia and therefore do not stand on the right side of the patient as he cannot see you.

Occasionally migrainous patients may have transient hemianopic defect with headache.

*Case History*: A 60-year-old male had an acute onset of right sided hemiplegia, recovered fairly well and was independently carrying on activities. Six months later he visited an ophthalmologist for inability to see with the right eye. He was operated for cataract in the right eye. However his vision did not improve. Subsequently neurological examination showed residual right hemianopia as a result of the previous stroke. It was not visual impairment.

*Diagnosis*: Right hemianopia.

*Message*: It is important to distinguish right sided visual loss due to eye problems from right hemianopic visual loss by simple bedside confrontation test.

*Bilateral cortical blindness*: Vertebrobasilar insufficiency causes transient or enduring cortical blindness, (pupils are normal and reactive with loss of vision). Both eyes are affected because the basilar artery which divides into posterior cerebral arteries supplies visual cortex on both sides.

## Oculomotor Nerve Palsy (III, IV and VI)

The eye movements are controlled by cranial nerves III, IV and VI. Isolated cranial nerve palsy III and VI are common but not IV.

### Testing of Eye Movements

Sit in front of the patient at a distance of three feet and ask the patient to follow the tip of your index finger with both eyes open. The finger is moved in all directions—horizontal, vertical initially slowly and then in quick succession. Normally the fast (saccades) and slow (pursuit) eye movements are well-coordinated. These are conjugate eye movements and are *disturbed in supranuclear pathway disorders*.

Individual eye movements are tested in all directions to assess the integrity of cranial nerves III, IV and VI. Diplopia is a manifestation of nuclear/infranuclear ocular palsy, resulting in misalignment of ocular movements. If the palsy is minimal, the images overlap and are *misinterpreted as blurring of vision*. This can be confirmed by closure of either eye when the blurring disappears. When the palsy is advanced, the images split resulting in double image (Table 9.5).

**Table 9.5: Causes of monocular diplopia.**
- Cataract
- Refractive error
- Opacity of media—cornea, lens
- Functional (malingering)

### Binocular Diplopia

III, IV and VI cranial nerve palsies.

### Isolated 3rd Cranial Nerve Palsy

Total paralysis causes ptosis and diplopia with paralysis of all ocular muscles except abduction (supplied by VI nerve) and dilated fixed pupil.

Third nerve palsy localization can be nuclear in the mid brain where it may be associated with long tract symptoms and signs—dysarthria, ataxia, hemiparesis or the lesion may be in the course of the third nerve due to a variety of causes like meningitis, tumors, cavernous sinus thrombosis, Tolosa-Hunt syndrome.

### In a Third Nerve Palsy when should Imaging of the Brain be done?

When 3rd nerve palsy is acute and is suggestive of ischemic infarct of nerve there is no need for MR imaging. However, if the 3rd nerve palsy is progressive or is associated with other symptoms like progressive headache, vomiting and difficulty in walking or paresis, suggestive of brain stem involvement, then 3rd nerve palsy is only a part of the story and to know the whole story further investigations including an MR brain is required (Table 9.6).

**Table 9.6: Localization of 3rd cranial nerve palsy.**

|  | Primary position | Diplopia | Pupils | Long tract signs (hemiparesis, ataxia) |
| --- | --- | --- | --- | --- |
| Supranuclear | Neutral | – | Normal | Yes |
| Nuclear | Squint | + | Dilated | Yes |
| Infranuclear | Squint | + | Dilated | – |
| Neuromuscular junction | Neutral/squint | + | Normal | – |
| Muscle | Neutral | – | Normal | – |

***Case History:*** A 60-year-old male, a known diabetic for five years, presented with acute onset of left sided ptosis of two days duration. He did not complain of diplopia simply because the ptosis was obstructing his vision. Clinical examination revealed medial rectus palsy in addition to left ptosis resulting in diplopia with sparing of the pupil. Additionally there was pain in the eye preceding the palsy. Diabetes is the commonest cause of isolated 3rd nerve palsy due to diabetic vascular complication affecting the nerve. This does not usually call for imaging of the brain.

**Diagnosis:** Left III nerve palsy.

**Message:** Painful third nerve palsy with sparing of pupil is typical of *diabetic cranial neuropathy* which spontaneously recovers over few weeks, with good control of diabetes. **Isolated fourth nerve palsy** is rare and is usually seen after a head injury. Typically the patient has diplopia while looking down, e.g. while going down the staircase.

**Isolated sixth nerve palsy** is the commonest cranial nerve palsy and majority of them have no specific cause (it is something like Bell's palsy of seventh nerve) probably due to microvascular infarct with or without diabetic state. Like Bell's palsy most of them recover over a period of a few weeks and the recovery can be speeded up by a short course of steroids.

**Multiple cranial nerve palsy** involving III, IV, VI nerves require proper investigations to find out the etiology.

**Supranuclear gaze palsy** is due to interruption of upper motor neuron fibers to oculomotor nuclei. As they involve both the eyes, *gaze palsy is without diplopia*. In a patient with stroke where it involves the frontal lobe, contralateral horizontal gaze palsy occurs with inability to look to the opposite side of the lesion with both the eyes. In pontine lesion, ipsilateral horizontal conjugate palsy is observed. Vertical gaze palsy is seen in mid brain lesions.

## Ocular Myopathy

In ocular myopathy, ocular muscles are symmetrically affected, hence *diplopia does not occur*. This is an important clinical clue. The pupil and pupillary reaction will be normal.

## Ptosis

Ptosis is drooping of the eye lid when the muscle levator palpebrae superioris is weak. The muscle is supplied by both sympathetic and parasympathetic innervation. This can be unilateral or bilateral, constant or fluctuating (Table 9.7).

The lesion can be due to:
a. Sympathetic paralysis
b. Parasympathetic paralysis in the 3rd cranial nerve from the nucleus to the cranial nerve—intracranial (diabetic 3rd nerve palsy) or intraorbital
c. Neuromuscular junction (myasthenia)
d. In the muscle (myopathy).

### Table 9.7: Anatomical localization for ptosis.

|  | Parasympathetic (cranial nerve III) | Sympathetic (Horner syndrome) | Neuromuscular junction (myasthenia) | Muscle (myopathy) |
|---|---|---|---|---|
| Pupil | Dilated | Constricted | Normal | Normal |
| Ocular palsy | Present | Absent | Present | Present |
| Diplopia | Present | Absent | Present (fluctuating) | Absent |
| Distribution | Unilateral/ occasionally bilateral | Unilateral | Bilateral | Bilateral |

### Unilateral Ptosis—Non-neurological Causes

One of the common causes of unilateral ptosis is aponeurotic rupture. Here the tendon insertion of levator palpebrae superioris is disrupted giving rise to *fixed unilateral ptosis* not obstructing the vision. More often it is friends or relatives who point out the ptosis. The patient is unaware of it. Diagnosis is confirmed by the high level of lid fold and thin muscle. It does not need any further investigation. It generally occurs in elderly following cataract surgery or due to contact lens or even rubbing of the eye. For cosmetic reasons, one may correct the mechanical ptosis.

### Unilateral Ptosis—Neurological Causes

Sympathetic innervation causes partial ptosis, which does not cover the pupil and hence vision is unaffected. The ptosis is usually observed by others. It is associated with sympathetic disturbances, like loss of sweating and a small pupil.

Unilateral ptosis due to parasympathetic involvement can cause partial or complete ptosis which means complete ptosis is always parasympathetic while partial ptosis can be due to sympathetic or para sympathetic involvement. The differentiation is by the size of the pupil—dilated in parasympathetic palsy and constricted in sympathetic palsy. In addition there will be evidence of paralysis of other ocular muscles supplied by third nerve.

### Bilateral Ptosis

*Ocular Myasthenia*

The commonest cause of fluctuating and asymmetric bilateral ptosis with diplopia is ocular myasthenia.

Mysthenia is muscle weakness and so the symptoms occur when the muscle is being used excessively. In the humans, levator palpebrae superioris is the only voluntary muscle which is kept active for 16 hours a day (if the person sleeps 8 hour a day), followed closely by ocular muscles. Hence myasthenia usually starts with ptosis and diplopia because of fatigue. As a person is reading a paper or watching TV gradually the words become blurred and the eyes close. After a brief rest he is back to normal again. Demonstration of fatigability is the key for diagnosis of ocular myasthenia. Ocular EMG is difficult to test and the response to neostigmine is inconsistent and hence it is entirely a clinical diagnosis. In the management also, neostigmine and pyridostigmine are less effective than the therapeutic response seen with steroids. If myasthenia is generalized it can be detected by EMG, otherwise it may be normal.

## Proptosis

Proptosis is the prominence of the eyeball, usually due to space occupying lesions like tumor, inflammatory granuloma mechanically pushing the eyeball out of the socket. The eyeball can be pushed out also when the *ocular muscles are swollen and weak* as in thyrotoxic ophthalmopathy. Normally ocular muscles rein in the eyeball into the orbit and when the muscles become weak it is pushed out. If proptosis is accompanied by chemosis (odema of the conjunctiva) it is due to associated venous obstruction either at the cavernous sinus or orbit levels (Table 9.8).

### Table 9.8: Differential diagnosis of proptosis.
- Dysthyroid exophthalmos—thyrotoxic ophthalmopathy—usually bilateral confirmed by elevated T4 levels
- Orbital cellulitis (proptosis, ophthalmoplegia, fever, chemosis)
- Orbital pseudotumor
- Lymphoma, space occupying lesion in orbit
- Cavernous sinus thrombosis

**Orbital Pseudotumor:** As the name implies all manifestations are like a tumor in the orbit pushing the eyeball out with or without compromising the vision. But when an imaging of the orbit is done there is no tumor, only swelling of the ocular muscles and granulomatous tissue. This responds very well to steroids.

*Case History:* A 35-year-old female had progressive left sided headache—orbital and retroorbital pain—with protrusion of eyeball with normal vision. Examination revealed left proptosis with striking chemosis with evidence of 3rd nerve palsy and additionally decreased pin sensation in the left trigeminal nerve ophthalmic division. This constellation of features is typical of *cavernous sinus thrombosis* (note to examine with pin the sensations over the left frontal area) and once this is confirmed the headache is due to trigeminal nerve involvement. MR brain confirmed the diagnosis.

*Diagnosis:* Cavernous sinus thrombosis.

**Message:** Involvement of vision localizes to orbit (Tables 9.9 and 9.10).

**Table 9.9:** Differential features of cavernous sinus thrombosis and Intra-orbital localization.

|  | Cavernous sinus thrombosis | Intraorbital localization |
|---|---|---|
| Structures involved | Internal carotid artery III, IV, V first division, VI cranial nerves | II III IV V – 1, VI Superior ophthalmic vein |
| Symptoms | Headache (V nerve 1st division) Proptosis, chemosis ocular palsies, dilated pupil | Pain in orbit, proptosis, **vision impairment,** restricted ocular movement |
| Causes | Infective, thrombosis | Pseudotumor, granuloma, abscess |

**Table 9.10:** Tolosa-Hunt syndrome (superior orbital fissure syndrome)—clinical features (painful ophthalmoplegia).

- Structures involved at superior orbital fissure III IV V-1 VI
- Symptoms: Retro-orbital pain, ophthalmoplegia
- Cause: Nonspecific inflammation of superior orbital tissue
- Treatment: Dramatic relief with high dose steroids, tapered over a month.

### Papilledema and Benign Intracranial Hypertension

- Papilledema is a sign of raised intracranial pressure with transient visual impairment (whenever the pressure raises further) with normal visual acuity. The visual impairment can be ascertained by perimetry which shows an enlarged blind spot and peripheral visual field constriction.
- If the imaging of the brain does not show any space occupying lesion one should investigate further for intracranial venous sinus thrombosis (MR venogram). When all these are normal we call *it benign intracranial hypertension* actually it is no more benign because it may eventually cause loss of vision. Hence the term "idiopathic intracranial hypertension" is appropriate. Lumbar puncture will show increased CSF pressure with normal values. This condition is typically seen in young obese females and the management consists of weight reduction and acetazolamide 250 mg to 1 gm a day to reduce the CSF production. One has to keep a tab on the vision and if visual failure sets in, optic sheath fenestration is recommended (Table 9.11).

**Table 9.11:** Differential diagnsois of blurring of optic disks.

|  | Optic neuritis | Papilledema | Drusen/pseudo-papilledema |
|---|---|---|---|
| Vision | Reduced | Normal | Normal |
| Pupillary reflex | Affected | Normal | Normal |
| Visual fields | Central scotoma | Enlarged blind spot | Normal |
| Assolciated findings | Blurring of disk margin | Hemorrhages | Nil |

# 10

# Syncope/Drop Attacks

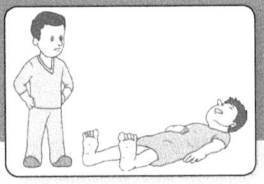

Syncope is the transient loss of consciousness with spontaneous recovery due to cerebral hypoperfusion. It is a self-limiting condition. The brain is dependent on continuous supply of blood which is pumped by the heart. When a person is standing or sitting, the heart has to pump the blood against the gravity to the overhead tank—the brain. Any condition which leads to transient decrease in cerebral blood flow to brain can cause syncope.

## CLINICAL MANIFESTATIONS

Presyncope warning symptoms before losing consciousness, which typically happens while the patient is standing, consists of blurring of vision, light headedness, dizziness, noises becoming distant, sweating and gradual slumping to the ground.

Syncope—here the patient may not remember the gradual fall to the ground but once he hits the ground, rapidly regains consciousness; there may be a few myoclonic jerks; if hypoxemia continues for longer period (as in cardiogenic syncope) there may be frank tonic-clonic seizures.

The common misdiagnosis is seizure, in view of transient loss of consciousness and jerking of limbs (Tables 10.1 and 10.2). Other associated symptoms distinguish the two, e.g. loud cry, sudden fall to the ground with or without injuries, tonic clonic movements, tongue bite, urinary incontinence. The person wakes up after several minutes with postictal confusion by which time he is usually shifted from the spot where he had fallen.

**Table 10.1: Differential diagnosis of transient loss of consciousness.**
- Seizure
- Syncope
- Vertebrobasilar insufficiency (associated brainstem features, e.g. diplopia, dysarthria, ataxia)
- Hypoglycemia (associated symptoms of hunger, sweating, palpitation, tremor)

**Table 10.2: Differential features of syncope/seizure.**

| | Syncope | Seizure |
|---|---|---|
| Trigger | Common (upright posture, sight of blood, needles) | Rare (flashing lights, hyperventilation) |
| Onset | Gradual sinking to ground | Usually sudden, abrupt fall |
| Duration | 10–30 seconds | 1–3 minutes |
| Tonic spasm | Uncommon | Common |
| Convulsive jerks | Common | Common |
| Injuries | Uncommon | Common |
| Incontinence | Uncommon | Common |
| Lateral tongue bite | Very rare | Common |
| Postictal confusion | Rare (e.g. wakes on floor where he had fallen) | Common (e.g. wakes in ambulance) |

## WHAT SHOULD BE THE MANAGEMENT?

The person should be made to lie down flat on the ground (no matter how dirty the floor is!). This position facilitates immediate resumption of blood supply to brain and rapid restoration of consciousness.

What usually happens is that the people around, try to prevent him from falling to the ground! Of course with good intention, and make him sit in a chair which continues the hypoxemia to the brain. This extended hypoxemia delays regaining of consciousness and may lead to frank seizures.

A person who has a history of recurrent presyncope/syncope should be instructed that as soon as he feels the symptoms of presyncope he should lie down flat. If that is not feasible at least he should sit down and bend his head to rest between the knees, to restore effective blood supply to brain. Types of syncopes are tabulated in (Table 10.3).

**Table 10.3: Types of syncope.**

a. Vasovagal syncope (Neurocardiogenic syncope)
b. Situational syncope—micturition, cough, deglutition, laughter
c. Cardiac syncope, e.g. Brady-and tachy-arrhythmias, aortic stenosis
d. Carotid sinus hypersensitivity
e. Orthostatic hypotension
   i. Due to antihypertensive drugs
   ii. Autonomic failure
      - Primary autonomic failure, e.g. multisystem atrophy (MSA). Postural orthostatic tachycardia syndrome (POTS)
      - Secondary to diabetic autonomic neuropathy, etc.

a. ***Vasovagal syncope:*** Is the commonest type of syncope where there is vasodilatation (due to sympathetic hypoactivity) and bradycardia (due to increased vagal activity)—the combination resulting in reduced cerebral blood flow.
**Trigger factors:** Prolonged standing, stuffy atmosphere, emotional upset, sight of blood.
The management is to lie down flat immediately, as soon as the pre-syncopal symptoms appear.
b. ***Situational syncope:*** Here a particular situation is a trigger factor for syncope.
**Micturition syncope:** Men have the privilege of passing urine in standing position and also have the privilege of having micturition syncope! This usually happens when the person wakes up in the middle of the night, goes to the toilet, half asleep and passes urine in the standing position. As the bladder is emptying syncope occurs, sometimes resulting in injury as the persons falls on the commode. **The management** is to avoid standing and passing urine, especially after waking up from sleep. I usually advise patients to get up gradually from the lying down position and once out of the bed to stand for several seconds shuffling the feet before proceeding to walk to the bathroom.
**Cough syncope:** As the name implies prolonged bouts of cough which results in increased intrathoracic pressure and reduced venous return can trigger a syncope. The management is the management of the cough!
c. ***Cardiogenic syncope:*** Due to Arrhythmias—bradyarrhythmias or tachyarrhythmias, sick sinus syndrome, valvular heart disease, aortic stenosis, left ventricular failure. In all these situations the cardiac output is reduced causing reduced cerebral blood flow and syncope. Where a cardiogenic syncope is suspected, cardiac consultation followed by ECG, Echocardiogram, Holter monitor, loop recorder may be required.

***Case History:*** A 75-year-old female hypertensive, diabetic presented with recurrent episodes of dizziness, followed by *gradual fall* to the ground unconscious terminating with tonic clonic seizure. She had 2-3 episodes/week for 3 months, and was on multiple antiepileptic drugs.

All investigations including Holter monitor were normal. The clinical diagnosis is probably cardiogenic syncope but not confirmed as yet. Fortunately on prolonged cardiac monitoring, she had two similar episodes, was diagnosed to have sick sinus syndrome. All her symptoms resolved after a cardiac pacemaker was introduced and antiepileptic drugs withdrawn.

***Diagnosis:*** Cardiogenic syncope.

***Message:*** If the patient does not experience the symptoms while the cardiac monitoring is on, the test is inconclusive. Until the event is captured on the ECG, diagnosis remains elusive. New onset seizures after the age of 60 years, cardiogenic causes (20-30%) to be considered.

**Management** is to treat the underlying cardiac cause.

d. **Carotid sinus hypersensitivity:** Tight fitting collars, head turning, carotid massage or palpation of carotid pulse may produce syncope—as a result of bradycardia, hypotension. Such persons should be advised to avoid precipitating factors.
e. **Orthostatic hypotension:** Typically syncope occurs as soon as the person changes the posture abruptly from supine to standing or sitting to standing. The diagnosis is made on the basis of fall in the blood pressure 20/10 mm Hg by change of posture. BP is recorded in resting supine position and in the standing position one minute and three minutes after standing.

Postural hypotension—Common cause is antihypertensive drugs and autonomic neuropathy as a result of diabetes; rarely due to primary autonomic failure, e.g. multisystem atrophy (MSA), Parkinson's disease.

Management consists of treating the underlying cause (adjustment of antihypertensive drugs). Symptomatic management in primary autonomic failure consists of increased fluid and salt intake, drugs like fludrocortisone (Salt retaining), midodrine (Vasoconstricting agent) may be added.

In addition patient education is helpful. The patient should be told to change the position gradually—to turn in bed gradually counting slowly up to seven, sit up gradually counting slowly up to seven, get out of bed and stand for a period counting slowly up to seven, once stabilized start moving. *Never get out of bed/chair suddenly and start walking.*

**Case History:** A 65-year-old female diabetic, hypertensive, had episodes of brief unconsciousness with spontaneous recovery—4–5 episodes in the previous 3 months. Detailed history revealed that all the episodes occurred when she was changing her posture from supine to standing or standing after prolonged sitting. Initial symptoms were darkening in front of the eyes, sweating and gradual fall to the ground, at times was able to sit down on her own. Within a minute or two she is conscious and able to get up and walk normally.

**Diagnosis:** Postural hypotension—syncope.

Symptoms are typical of postural syncope and the diagnosis is entirely on the history. Repeated examination of blood pressure in supine and standing positions, immediately and 3 minutes later was informative with drop in blood pressure *reproducing the symptoms*. A tilt table test can also contribute to the diagnosis. In this case as the patient happens to be doctor's mother all possible investigations including MR brain, MR angiogram, carotid Doppler and EEG were done. Carotid Doppler showed 70% stenosis on the right side and MR brain showed a few lacunar infarcts. She was put on aspirin, clopidogrel and atorvastatin.

Carotid stenosis has *nothing to do with her syncopal episodes*. Syncope is always due to global hypoperfusion and carotid stenosis produces focal deficit, e.g. hemiparesis. In this case both carotid stenosis and lacunar infarcts are incidental which is seen in a large number of senior citizens. There is no role for antiplatelet drugs and statins as this is not a transient ischemic attack.

# CHAPTER 11

# Seizure/Epilepsy

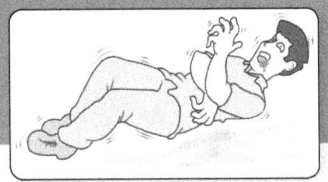

Seizures, fits, convulsions are descriptive terms emphasizing on the clonic movements of limbs and occur due to a variety of conditions, e.g. hypoglycemia, hepatic dysfunction, renal dysfunction, etc.

*Epilepsy is defined as two or more unprovoked seizures.* Even though there are some recent modifications in the definition, this definition is very practical and easy to implement.

Epilepsy is a common neurological disorder affecting almost 1% of the population. The good news about epilepsy is that it is eminently treatable in 70-75% and in the remaining 25-30%, when pharmacotherapy fails, surgical treatment is an option with good results. Not only that, a few seizures occurring over a short period of six months to a year can spontaneously disappear in about 20%! The medication can be withdrawn after 2-5 years of seizure free period (two years for GTCS and 5 years for CPS). The person with epilepsy is totally normal between the two attacks and can do everything a normal person can do including education, sports, jobs, computer, TV, marriage, pregnancy, children, breastfeeding and there are no diet restrictions! Even driving and swimming is allowed after a seizure free period of 1-2 years.

With so much of good news why is it that a diagnosis of epilepsy devastates the patient and the entire family? It is simply because of myths, misunderstandings and stigma attached to epilepsy which have been carried down the ages—more than five thousand years!

## EPILEPSY—OVERDIAGNOSED

Epilepsy in clinical practice is an *overdiagnosed* condition. When a person falls down and is unconscious for a very brief period—as it happens in syncope, it is mistakenly diagnosed as epilepsy with all its social consequences and unnecessary prolonged treatment. The next common wrong diagnosis is when a person has convulsive movements with "unconsciousness" as seen in a non-epileptic attack disorder (psychogenic seizures, hysterical seizures). This means that epilepsy should be clearly differentiated from syncope and non epileptic attack disorder.

## EPILEPSY—DIAGNOSTIC STEPS

*Step 1*: Is it a seizure?
*Step 2*: Is the seizure provoked or unprovoked?
*Step 3*: Single/two or more seizures?
*Step 4*: Type of epilepsy?

### Step 1: Is it a seizure?

Make sure the clinical presentation is seizure and differentiate it from syncope or non-epileptic attack disorder (Tables 11.1 and 11.2).

**Table 11.1: Epilepsy vs syncope.**

| Clinical features | Epilepsy | Syncope |
|---|---|---|
| Onset | Sudden | Gradual fall |
| Precipitating factors | None | Standing for long time |
| Sweating | - | + |
| Tongue bite | +/- | - |
| Injury | +/- | - |
| Postictal confusion | + | - |
| Duration | Several minutes | Several seconds |

For more details about syncope see Chapter 9.

**Table 11.2: Epilepsy vs non-epileptic attack.**

| | Epilepsy | Non-epileptic attack (functional/psychogenic) |
|---|---|---|
| Onset | Sudden | Gradual |
| Seizure | Rhythmic tonic-clonic | Bizarre movement of limbs, head No set pattern |
| Urinary incontinence | May occur | No |
| Tongue bite | Common | No |
| Duration | One to two minutes | Prolonged—sometimes hours |
| Eyes | Open | Closed |
| Attack pattern | Stereotype | Variable |

***Case History:*** A 12-year-old male had four episodes of unconsciousness in school and one episode at home. He complains of giddiness and then lies down unresponsive for 10–15 minutes, no tonic-clonic seizures. EEG showed non-specific changes. He was diagnosed to have epilepsy and started on levetiracetam. As the history was not suggestive of epilepsy, he was referred to a neuropsychologist for evaluation. The detailed history revealed that his class teacher was demanding the food brought by him in the lunchbox leaving him hungry. Also, the teacher was demanding that he should bring sweets and choicest dishes. One day he was so hungry, he felt weak and fell down. The teacher got scared and allowed him to take his food. This resulted in his episodes of "unconsciousness" to make sure that his food is not taken by the teacher. When asked why he did not tell his parents, he said that he was afraid the teacher may get angry and punish him. The parents and the boy were counseled and the antiepileptic drug withdrawn.

*Diagnosis*: Non-epileptic attack disorder.

*Case History*: A 10-year-old female presented with left simple partial motor seizures affecting the left upper limb, at times progressing to generalized tonic-clonic seizures due to right parietal solitary ring enhancing lesion. The seizures abated and the granuloma resolved. Three months later she presented with recurrent left partial motor seizures which continued in spite of the CT showing a healed granuloma and increasing the antiepileptic drug dosage. I reviewed my diagnosis. Further history revealed that the seizures were prolonged, sometimes lasting for 30–45 minutes occurring in the morning especially at the time of going to school. Video EEG confirmed that it was non-epileptic events. The antiepileptic drugs were tapered off and patient was referred to a psychiatrist.

*Diagnosis*: Non-epileptic attack disorder.

**Message:** Whenever the pattern of seizures change, particularly in duration, one should think of functional/psychogenic causes.

### Step 2: Is the seizure provoked or unprovoked?

The cerebral cortex which is the anatomical substrate for generating epileptic discharges can be provoked by a variety of physiological disturbances or structural involvement of the brain (Table 11.3).

**Table 11.3: Provoked seizures.**

- *Systemic causes*—Febrile seizure
- Metabolic Encephalopathy, e.g. Hepatic, renal dysfunction
- Electrolyte imbalance (Hypo, hypernatremia)
- *Cerebral causes*—Meningoencephalitis
- Head injury, stroke

Provoked seizures due to physiological disturbances *do not require* continuation of antiepileptic drugs at discharge from hospital. For example, the patient may be admitted with frequent seizures and then found to have hypoglycemia/hyponatremia for which AEDs are given for symptomatic control of seizures. Once the underlying cause is addressed and seizures stop, at discharge the AEDs too should be stopped. In provoked seizures due to structural lesion of the brain, e.g. viral encephalitis, the seizures are symptomatically controlled and the AEDs continued for the next three months after discharge from the hospital. As a result of structural damage, a few patients may continue to have seizures. However at the time of three months follow-up if the patient is seizure free then the *AED can be withdrawn*. Unfortunately in clinical practice I see that in a large number of patients with provoked seizures, AEDs are continued for 3–5 years with a label of epilepsy!

*Remember provoked seizures are not epilepsy.*

### Step 3: Single/two or more seizures?

Having made sure that the patient had a seizure which was unprovoked, the next question is, whether it is the first seizure? The definition of epilepsy says "two or more unprovoked seizures." The treatment of epilepsy is to prevent the next seizure. So what are the chances of developing the next seizure after the first seizure? Statistics show that it may vary from 30–70%. Generally we do not start AEDs after the first seizure. If there is any evidence of "brain damage" like head injury, cerebral palsy or stroke, with the chances of recurrence being high, AEDs are started.

### Step 4: Type of Epilepsy?

Having fulfilled the definition of "two or more unprovoked seizures" now the diagnosis of epilepsy is established. The next step is to find out the type of epilepsy. It is important to identify the type of epilepsy because the choice of AED depends on the type of epilepsy. The classification of epilepsy is very complicated; however from the practice point of view, for a non-neurologist the following classification is practical (Table 11.4).

**Table 11.4: Classification of epilepsy.**
- Generalized seizures—Tonic-clonic seizures, absences, myoclonic
- Partial seizure—Simple—Sensory, motor Complex
- Partial becoming generalized

The clinical features of various types of epilepsies are as under (Tables 11.5 to 11.8):

**Table 11.5: Clinical features—generalized tonic-clonic seizures (GTCS).**
- Sudden onset, cry
- Unconscious, tonic-clonic movements
- Tongue bite, incontinence
- Postictal sleep, headache, vomiting

**Table 11.6: Clinical features—absences.**
- Occurs in children (5–15 years)
- Abrupt onset, blinking 3 times/second
- Unaware
- Lasts for few seconds
- Several attacks/day
- No postictal confusion
- Easily elicited by hyperventilation

#### Table 11.7: Clinical features—Juvenile myoclonic epilepsy (JME).

- Onset in adolescence
- Myoclonic jerks of upper limb, at times lower limbs
- Occurs in clusters, usually in the first two hours after waking
- Precipitated by lack of sleep

#### Table 11.8: Clinical features—complex partial seizure (CPS).

- Sudden onset
- Abdominal discomfort
- Staring unresponsive, chewing, champing movements, automatism
- Brief postictal confusion

Whenever a patient presents with GTCS it is mandatory to ask whether the patient has CPS/absence/JME, to properly classify the type of epilepsy and to choose the appropriate drug. Patient may come with GTCS and you start on CBZ, but the seizures continue to worsen. When you ask for a detailed history the patient reports of also having infrequent myoclonic jerks; now the diagnosis changes from GTCS to JME, the drug of choice being VPA. In fact, CBZ increases the seizures in JME. This clearly illustrates the need for classifying the type of epilepsy by spending time on history.

*Hot water epilepsy* — is a reflex epilepsy (Table 11.9).

#### Table 11.9: Clinical features—hot water epilepsy.

- Reflex epilepsy occurring *while* hot water is poured on the head
- Features of complex partial seizure infrequently terminating in GTCS
- Treatment: Avoid hot water head bath, can use hot water for rest of the body
- When head bath is required Clobazam 10 mg to be given one hour before bath

***What are the investigations for confirming the diagnosis of epilepsy?*** Infact none! The diagnosis of epilepsy is entirely clinical and is based on the history from the patient and from the observer. The eye witness account of the event is the deciding factor for diagnosis, e.g. patient may say that he felt giddy, fell down and immediately got up—this may mean syncope. However the history from the observer is different, who says that the patient fell down abruptly, had tonic-clonic seizures and postictal confusion—all of which the patient is unaware of and therefore the patient thinks that he immediately got up after the fall. Recording the attack on mobile video and showing it to doctor will be of immense help to make a proper diagnosis.

***What is EEG for?*** EEG records the electrical activity of the brain (encephalon). As epilepsy is periodic, so also the abnormal electrical discharges occur at random and the chances of picking up this abnormality in the routine EEG recording is only about 40%. So a normal EEG does not rule out epilepsy. On the other hand EEG may show non-specific electrical abnormalities like non-specific ST-T changes. The role of EEG is to identify the type of epilepsy, e.g. a patient may present with GTCS, the detailed history does not reveal any myoclonic jerks, however the EEG may show poly spike wave discharges suggestive of JME. The diagnosis is now changed from GTCS to JME with the help of EEG. The EEG can suggest the type of epilepsy, e.g. CPS, JME and absences.

### What is the role of imaging (CT/MR Brain)?

Imaging only gives us the structural abnormality. Epilepsy being a functional disturbance, imaging will be normal in great majority.

Imaging in epilepsy is done *not for diagnosis* of epilepsy but to look for symptomatic causes like brain tumor, brain TB, etc. (Figs. 11.1 to 11.3) (Table 11.10).

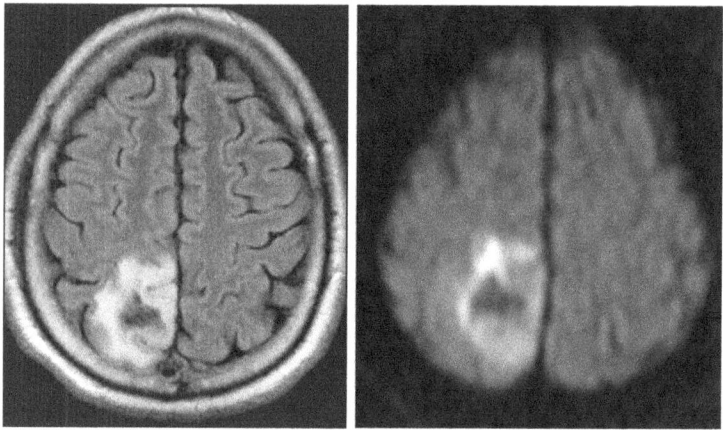

**Fig. 11.1:** MR brain—right parietal glioma.

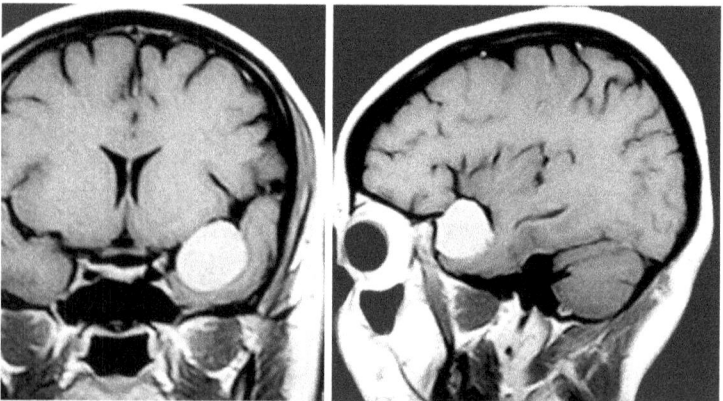

**Fig. 11.2:** MR brain—left temporal meningioma.

Seizure/Epilepsy

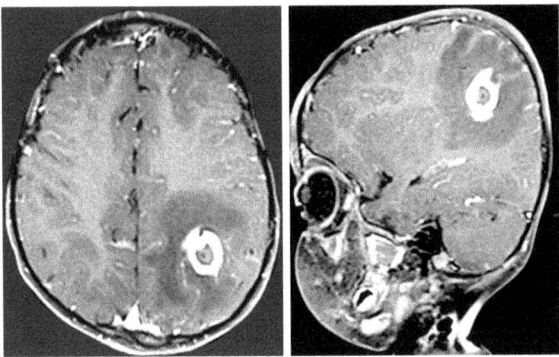

Fig. 11.3: MR brain—left parietal tuberculoma.

**Table 11.10: Indications for imaging in epilepsy.**
- Epilepsy + any other neurologic symptoms/signs, e.g. diplopia, hemiparesis, dysarthria, personality changes, papilloedema
- Epilepsy starting after the age of 35 years
- Drug resistant epilepsy

Imaging is necessary only when symptomatic epilepsy is thought of, i.e. epilepsy + any other neurological symptom (diplopia, dysarthria, hemiparesis, visual blurring, progressive headache, personality changes, memory impairment) or signs, e.g. papilloedema.

Solitary cysticercus lesion resulting in a flurry of partial/generalized seizures is a fairly common cause of symptomatic epilepsy in our country (Fig. 11.4). Postictal paresis is observed in some patients.

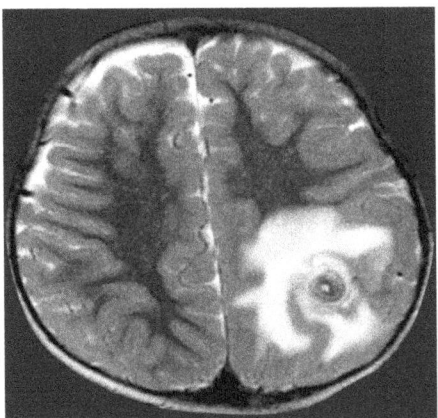

Fig. 11.4: MR brain—left parietal neurocysticercosis.

*Case History*: A 25-year-old male had new onset generalized seizures followed by inability to lift the upper limb which initially was thought as postictal paresis. MR brain scan was normal. The paresis "persisted" even on the second day.

Examination showed normal motor power—grip and elbow, but patient was unable to lift the left upper limb at shoulder. In postictal paresis *distal muscles are affected first* and the most. Here the distal muscles were normal and the passive movement of the shoulder was painful.

**Diagnosis** is dislocation of the shoulder joint and not postictal paresis.

**Message**: Immediately after a seizure, inability to move the upper limb can be due to paresis or shoulder dislocation which can be easily differentiated by the passive movement of the shoulder which is painful with well preserved strength of the distal muscles.

Other reasons for doing an imaging are late onset epilepsy, i.e. seizures occurring after the age of 35 years simply because symptomatic seizures are more common in this age group.

In medically refractory epilepsy MR scan—"epilepsy protocol" will look for surgically remediable lesions, e.g. mesial temporal sclerosis, developmental cortical anomalies.

### Which Imaging?

Obviously the imaging of choice is MR scan because of its ability to delineate the structure of brain in great detail, e.g. medial temporal sclerosis—a common cause in complex partial seizures, cortical developmental anomalies—a common cause in pediatric and adolescent intractable seizures, DNET tumors, cavernoma, glioma etc.

### Which AED to start?

In the last few years a number of newer AEDs have flooded the market. In general, the newer AEDs and the older AEDs are equally effective in controlling the seizures. However, the newer AEDs have lesser side-effects but are more expensive. The first choice should be an appropriate AED from among the older AEDs (Table 11.11).

| Table 11.11: Choice of AED. | | |
| --- | --- | --- |
| *Seizure type* | *First line* | *Second line* |
| Tonic-clonic seizures | PB, PHT, CBZ, VPA | OXC, LTG, LEV |
| Juvenile myoclonic epilepsy | VPA, CLZ | LTG |
| Complex partial seizures | CBZ, PHT | OXC, LTG, LEV |
| Simple partial seizures | PHT, CBZ, PB | VPA, OXC |
| Absences | VPA, ESM | LTG |
| Clobazam is an excellent add on drug for CPS and GTCS | | |

*Always start* with a small dose and gradually increase the dosage, if the seizures keep recurring, to the required dose. If one AED is not able to control the seizures then try the next appropriate AED or add a second drug. Always consider the cost of the AED as the medicines have to be taken over a period of 2-5 years. Newer AEDs and the indications are mentioned in Tables 11.12 and 11.13.

### Table 11.12: Newer AED.

- Oxcarbazepine
- Levetiracetam
- Lamotrigine
- Topiramate
- Lacosamide
- Zonisamide
- Vigabatrin

### Table 11.13: Indication for newer AED.

- Failure of first line drugs—as an add on drug
- Intolerance/allergy to first line drugs

#### When to withdraw AED?

AED is withdrawn by trial and error and more trials and more errors! It is now accepted that after a two year seizure free period for GTCS and a five year seizure free period for CPS one can start tapering off the AED. One should ensure that there are no big attacks (GTCS) and small attacks (CPS, MJ) before the AED is withdrawn. The drugs are never stopped abruptly but tapered off—one tablet every 2-3 months.

In JME it is said that the treatment is for an indefinite period. However one can attempt to withdraw the AED after 5 years and if there is recurrence (which is high), the AED should be reintroduced.

#### Risk of Recurrence

The recurrence can occur while the drug is being withdrawn or within six to twelve months after stopping the drug. The risk is less in GTCS (5-10%) than in CPS (25-30%) and JME (80-90%). If there is recurrence, the drug is reintroduced in the last effective dose and continued for another 2-3 years and an attempt is once again made to withdraw the drug.

*Antiepileptic drug assay*—is an over-used and much abused investigation. If the seizures are well controlled there is no need to increase or decrease the dosage irrespective of the laboratory report. AED levels are useful when a patient is on polytherapy, with toxic side-effects, to know which drug is in the toxic range. Similarly, AED levels can check the compliance when the patient says he is taking medicine regularly, but continues to have seizures.

***Clobazam*** is a fast acting oral antiepileptic drug used as bridge therapy and intermittently in "situation related seizures" like febrile seizures, hot water epilepsy, catamenial epilepsy and as a prophylactic in sleep deprived states like international travel and honeymoon period!

### Epilepsy and Social Aspects

It is easier to treat seizures in a patient with epilepsy but very difficult to address the social implications. In other illnesses like hypertension and diabetes the patient and immediate family members are educated in the management of the disease. In epilepsy not only the patient and the family members but the entire society needs to be educated! Out of ignorance and stigma attached to epilepsy a person with epilepsy even when the seizures are very well controlled, is denied admission to school, college, is discriminated in employment, sports, marriage, pregnancy and recreational activities. At home unnecessary restrictions are imposed on diet, TV, computer, etc. It is the responsibility of the physician to educate the patient and the family.

P.S. For more detailed information the reader is referred to the Book "Manual of Epilepsy—Medical Management and Social Aspects" by Dr HV Srinivas.

# CHAPTER 12

# Difficulty to Talk

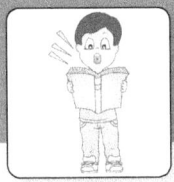

**Doctor, I am not able to talk as I used to**

When a patient complains of difficulty in talking it is important to distinguish language disorder (dysphasia) from articulation disorder (dysarthria) (Tables 12.1 and 12.2).

**In Dysphasia** there is difficulty to construct a sentence, to write, to understand spoken/written words.

The lesion is specifically in the dominant hemisphere—the perisylvian area.

**In Dysarthria** language production is normal, but the delivery mechanism is affected, i.e. the sentence will be well constructed but the smooth flow will be interrupted. This is due to weakness/incoordination of muscles of articulation (e.g. tongue, palate, facial muscles). It is obvious that in dysarthria the patient can understand spoken and written words and can also write with either hand.

## HOW TO TEST THE LANGUAGE

Language has four components: Two motor or expressive and two sensory or receptive.

### Motor (Expressive)

- **Spoken:** Observe the way the person speaks, full sentence or only a few words.
- **Written:** Even if the patient has paralysis of the right side and is unable to hold the pen in the right hand, if the language functions are intact one can still write with the left hand. If unable to write then it is a sign of expressive aphasia.

### Sensory (Receptive)

- **Verbal instruction:** The patient is able to understand words spoken to him/her—one should say simple requests like "close your eyes, put out your tongue, touch your left ear" and these instructions must be given with a *straight face without mimicking. Often* the relatives will mimic the requests by putting out the tongue, closing the eyes and asking the patient to imitate—this is not verbal understanding, it becomes a visual cue.

❑ **Written instruction:** The patient is able to understand the written words (if he is literate). The same instructions mentioned above can be written and shown to the patient and see whether he can understand and follow them.

*A typical example of dysphasia is as follows:*

**Normal speech:** When the husband wants to have a cup of coffee he tells his wife "My dear darling, will you be kind enough to prepare a cup of coffee for me which I would love to have from you".

**In Dysphasia:** Instead of this full sentence which cannot be formulated the patient will look at his wife and say "Coffee". This one word conveys the entire message. This is also known as a "telegraphic language" where you use minimum words to convey the message.

(Of course this telegraphic language can also happen normally after a few years of marriage !!).

In **dysarthria** the above sentence is spoken completely but may not be understandable because of the pronunciation/articulation defect.

Usually dysarthria is part of a neurological illness "Tell me who your friend is and I will tell you who you are" holds good here. If dysarthria is associated with other cerebellar features or extrapyramidal features then it is obvious that articulation is simultaneously affected.

**Table 12.1: Aphasia—types.**

| Types | Speech output | Comprehension |
|---|---|---|
| Broca's | Non-fluent | Good |
| Wernicke's | Fluent | Poor |
| Global | Non-fluent | Poor |

**Table 12.2: Differential features of dysphasia and dysarthria.**

| Dysphasia (Language dysfunction) | Dysarthria (Difficulty in articulation) |
|---|---|
| Motor—Inability to talk, inability to write | Able to form sentences but pronunciation is skewed |
| Sensory—Inability to understand spoken and written words | Able to write and understand spoken and written words |
| Lesion—Perisylvian area of dominant hemisphere | **Lesions**<br>LMN—Wasting tongue<br>UMN—Spastic tongue<br>Cerebellar—Incoordination<br>Extrapyramidal—Slow movement<br>Abnormal movements—Dyskinesia, dystonia<br>Neuromuscular dysfunction—Myasthenia<br>Muscle—Myopathy |
| Associated features—Right hemiparesis | Symptoms related to any one of the above systems |

**Case History:** A 45-year-old female was referred for second opinion with a diagnosis of "bulbar motor neuron disease". She had difficulty in talking of one and half years duration with wasting of tongue. EMG of the tongue showed fibrillation potentials. Review of the history showed that she had 'sudden' onset of difficulty in talking which has remained stable. Examination showed isolated unilateral tongue atrophy with fasciculation

*Step 1*: Neurological deficit—Left XII nerve LMN palsy.

*Step 2*: Anatomical localization—Isolated left XII cranial nerve. There were no symptoms suggestive of brainstem involvement at the onset, like ataxia or hemiparesis.

*Step 3*: Pathological diagnosis—Acute onset, non-progressive, vascular/demyelination.

*Step 4*: Etiological diagnosis—Isolated cranial nerve palsy—cause ischemic/inflammatory demyelination.

**Diagnosis:** Isolated left XII cranial nerve palsy.

**Message:** It is the history which differentiated an innocuous isolated XII nerve palsy from moribund "bulbar motor neuron disease". This patient met me 10 years later with partial improvement in speech and thanked me for changing the diagnosis from MND, as she was devastated with the diagnosis of MND and the internet information on this.

# CHAPTER 13

# Difficulty to Write

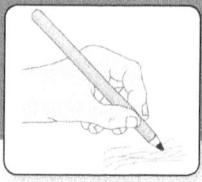

**Doctor, I have difficulty to write**

The first question to the patient is whether the difficulty is *exclusively* for writing or also for other activities with the hand like mixing food, eating, brushing, shaving, etc. The latter is part of motor weakness affecting the hand which can be seen in several situations like UMN paresis, LMN paresis, Parkinson's disease, etc.

**Exclusive** difficulty in writing is a "task specific" condition and occurs due to:

a. **Focal dystonia:** Also known as "writer's cramp". As the person holds the pen and starts writing there is excessive contraction of muscles of forearm which presses the pen firmly on the paper. The patient complains of pain in the forearm and the grip on the pen loosens. This is an extrapyramidal disorder and responds marginally to medication with anticholinergic drugs (trihexyphenidyl). The more effective treatment is Botox injection to the muscles which are undergoing spasm, and this gives relief for few months. As this procedure is expensive and requires to be taken periodically, I usually suggest to the patient to start practicing writing with the left hand which is very cost effective! Nowadays people use a pen very occasionally for writing and even signing the cheques is passe with digitalization. So, if the patient's daily activities are unaffected there is no need to give any treatment!

b. **Writing tremor:** Here the difficulty in writing is due to tremors of the hands which are *exclusive* to writing only. The management consists of prescribing Propranolol in adequate doses. The alternative drug is Primidone.

# 14
# Gait Imbalance

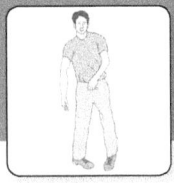

Gait disorders and imbalance in walking is common in elderly resulting in falls and injuries. Normal walking and maintaining the balance while walking are due to the following inputs:
- Sensory inputs to brain: The sensory inputs of position of legs consist of visual, proprioceptive receiving position and joint senses and muscle spindles.
- Coordinated movements of legs: Cerebellar.
- Additional factors: Vestibular, cognition.
- Motor power in lower limbs to execute the movement.

When a person presents with difficulty to walk the problem can be neurological or non-neurological (Table 14.1). The common non-neurological conditions are osteoarthritis of the knee or hip where the pain in that particular joint is the limiting factor.

### Table 14.1: Types of gait disorder.
- Wide based gait—sensory ataxia, cerebellar ataxia, cautious gait
- Narrow based gait—Parkinson's disease
- Waddling gait—proximal muscle weakness
- Circumduction gait—spastic gait

Once the non-neurological causes are excluded then the neurological causes can be broadly divided into—motor weakness, stiffness of limbs and incoordination (Table 14.2).

### Table 14.2: Difficulty in walking—causes.

| I. Motor weakness | II. Stiffness of limbs | III. Incoordination (ataxia) | IV. Psychological |
|---|---|---|---|
| UMN | UMN (Spasticity) | Cerebellar | Phobic disorder |
| LMN (Anterior horn cell, root, plexus peripheral nerves) | Extrapyramidal (Rigidity) | Sensory (Post column, Peripheral nerve) | Anxiety |
| Neuromuscular junction (myasthenia) | Muscle (Myotonia) | Vestibular | |
| | Dystonia | | |
| Muscle (myopathy) | Stiff-person syndrome | | |

Observe the gait while the patient is walking.

The first step is to identify which of the above is responsible for the difficulty in walking.

## MOTOR WEAKNESS

Clinical neurological examination will reveal reduced strength of muscles confirming the presence of motor weakness. This has to be further analyzed whether it is due to UMN (Hypertonia, brisk reflexes, plantar extensor), LMN (hypotonia, absent tendon reflexes), myopathy (Proximal muscles more affected than distal) or myasthenia (fatigability, fluctuating motor weakness).

Motor weakness is discussed in **Chapter 15.**

## STIFFNESS

Stiffness as a cause of difficulty in walking is discussed in **Chapter 15.**

## ATAXIA

Some patients have good power in the limbs; they can kick the football but are unable to walk steadily. Clinical examination reveals normal motor power and supple limbs but yet they are unable to walk due to incoordination of lower limbs. Watching the patient getting out of chair, walking briskly, taking a sudden turn gives good functional assessment of balance.

Ataxia can be further divided into (Table 14.3):
i. Cerebellar ataxia
ii. Sensory ataxia
iii. Vestibular ataxia.

To identify which one is responsible follow the dictum "Tell me who your friend is and I will tell you who you are".

In sensory ataxia the associated sensory symptoms are tingling, numbness and paresthesia. In cerebellar ataxia associated symptoms are ataxia in upper limbs and speech involvement. In vestibular ataxia there are distinct vestibular symptoms with vertigo and vomiting.

If a patient with ataxia has speech involvement it is diagnostic of cerebellar ataxia. If there is associated upper limb involvement it is usually cerebellar. Differential diagnosis is wide open between cerebellar, sensory, and vestibular if there is ataxia only in the lower limbs.

## Table 14.3: Gait ataxia—types.

| Types | Anatomical substrate | Associated features | Investigations |
|---|---|---|---|
| Cerebellar | ❏ Cerebellum or<br>❏ Cerebellar connections in brainstem | Dysarthria hypotonia, hyporeflexia, dysmetria, multidirectional nystagmus | MR brain |
| Sensory | Loss of proprioception<br>❏ Sensory neuropathy<br>❏ Sensory radiculopathy<br>❏ Posterior columns in spinal cord | Loss of position, vibration sense<br>Romberg +ve<br>Peripheral neuropathy<br><br>Associated UMN signs of spinal cord | <br><br><br>NCV<br><br>MR spinal cord |
| Vestibular | ❏ Peripheral (vestibular nerve, labyrinth)<br>❏ Central (brainstem) | Vomiting, sweating<br><br>Diplopia, dysarthria<br>Dysphagia | MR brain |

### Cerebellar Ataxia

The cerebellar gait is wide based and there is a tendency to fall while turning, may or may not be accompanied by other cerebellar features like dysarthria and upper limb incoordination (Table 14.4).

## Table 14.4: Cerebellar ataxia—treatable conditions.

| | |
|---|---|
| Drug Induced | Phenytoin, Carbamazepine, Lithium |
| Toxic | Alcohol |
| Nutritional | Vit B12, Vit B1 deficiency |
| Infection | Viral infections |
| Endocrine | Hypothyroidism |
| Demyelination | MS, ADEM |
| Vascular | Ischemic, Hemorrhagic stroke |
| Tumors | Benign, primary, secondaries |

Cerebellar atrophy (Fig. 14.1) and Cerebellar malignant tumor (Fig. 14.2) are non-treatable or partially treatable conditions.

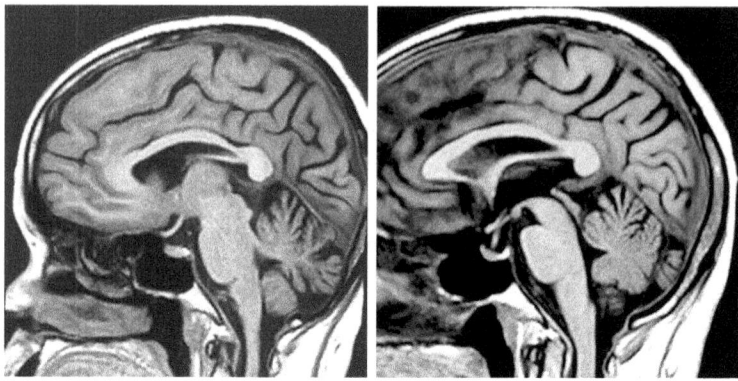

Fig. 14.1: Cerebellar atrophy.

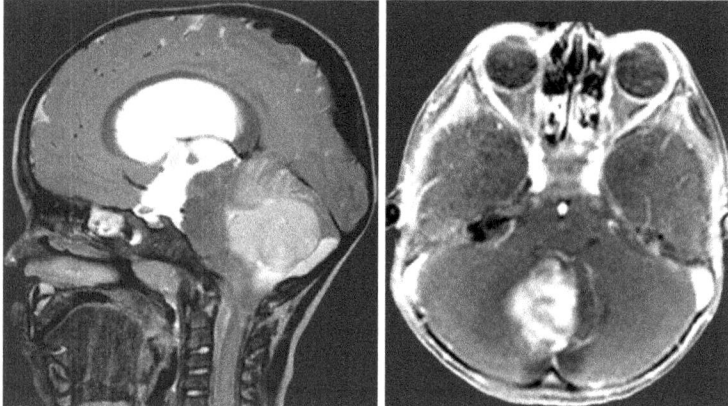

Fig. 14.2: Cerebellar tumor.

***Case History:*** A 65-year-old female presented with new onset generalized seizures with minimal right hemiparesis (due to left cerebral infarction). She recovered from hemiparesis within a week and was able to walk normally. However within the next week she again developed difficulty in walking which gradually increased. A repeat MR was done which was non-contributory. When examined she had gait ataxia and was on Phenytoin 100 mg 3 times a day. The drug was stopped for two days and reintroduced in a smaller dose. Gait ataxia disappeared.

Phenytoin 100 mg tds when prescribed to senior citizens very frequently leads to cerebellar ataxia. The dose should start with 100 mg and increased to 200 mg after ten days.

***Diagnosis:*** Phenytoin toxicity.

## Sensory Ataxia

There is gait imbalance due to absence of sensory inputs from the periphery. The person looks down while walking to see where his feet are. The ataxia worsens with eye closure. Typically it happens while walking in the dark or while closing the eyes while washing face (wash basin phenomena). Stable with eyes open and feet together, unstable to the extent of falling when eyes are closed is a sign of sensory ataxia (Rhomberg's sign). Some amount of instability is not sufficient for Romberg's sign but instability to the extent of falling is important (Table 14.5).

**Table 14.5: Sensory ataxia—treatable conditions.**
- AIDP/CIDP
- MS
- Cervical spondylotic myelopathy
- Vit B12 deficiency
- Peripheral neuropathy, e.g. Diabetic.

*Case History*: A 45-year-old male presented with three days history of rapidly progressive gait imbalance, so much so that after one or two steps he used to fall down. The entry for diagnosis is "gait ataxia" affecting only lower limbs which means it could be due to any of the three conditions—vestibular, (vestibular gait disorder follows an episode of vestibular dysfunction, e.g. vertigo, vomiting), sensory ataxia and cerebellar.

*Step 1*: *Neurological deficit*—Clinical examination showed gross posterior column dysfunction (absent vibration, position sense in the lower limbs with Romberg's sign positive, absent tendon reflexes in both knee and ankle).

*Step 2*: *Anatomical localization*—Posterior column sensation involvement in the root (sensory radiculopathy) or in the spinal cord. There was no evidence of bladder involvement or UMN signs, which if present could have localized clinically to spinal cord.

*Investigation for anatomical localization*—Nerve conduction studies showed totally normal sensory, peripheral as well as root motor fibers. Hence the next investigation asked for was spinal cord and MR thoracic spine both plain and contrast. This showed a long segment demyelinating lesion from C2 to D1 specifically affecting the posterior columns.

*Step 3*: *Pathological diagnosis*—Acute demyelination of cervical cord.

*Step 4*: *Etiological diagnosis*—Probably immune mediated- MS or NMO—to investigate further. Patient improved gradually after pulse therapy with methylprednisolone.

*Diagnosis*: Thoracic cord demyelination.

### Vestibular Ataxia

Associated with vestibular dysfunction, e.g. vomiting, vertigo.

*Case History*: A 35-year-old male presented with acute onset of vertigo, vomiting, gait ataxia, though vomiting resolved two days later, gait ataxia continued for another week.

*Diagnosis*: Acute vestibular neuronitis.

### "Psychogenic" Ataxia

The gait is variable, erratic, as though walking on ice but the person never falls. Neurological examination is unremarkable, though the patient feels unsteady while walking. Anxiety and depression are accompanying features. There may be unsteadiness in situations like crossing the road or walking on the street, but is quite comfortable to walk while holding the hand of a child (psychological support). Best managed with anxiolytics and counseling.

## MISCELLANEOUS GAIT DISORDERS

### Cautious Gait

Very common in elderly and is also non-specific in the sense that it does not represent any one particular neurological condition. The walking is very slow, unsteady, with excessive fear of falling. The lack of confidence may be multifactorial like knee joint pain, peripheral sensory neuropathy, hearing impairment, visual impairment, cognitive impairment, etc. Each factor by itself may not be severe enough but a combination of several factors leads to this condition. The best recommend way of management is using a walking stick preferably with three legs to reduce the risk of a fall and fracture of neck of femur. It is amazing how senior citizens resist using a walking stick, as they feel extreme loss of self esteem!

In addition, external factors can contribute to the falls, e.g. uneven flooring, poor lighting.

**Postural imbalance** is usually due to axial rigidity as in extra pyramidal disorder. This causes fall to the ground in a *fully conscious state*. The diagnosis is easy in cases of Parkinson's disease where axial rigidity is but one manifestation of the entire clinical spectrum of tremors/rigidity. However in cases of progressive supranuclear palsy, axial rigidity and frequent falls are the presenting manifestations. When suspected one should carefully examine vertical eye movements especially, the downward movement which is lost. One clinical clue is they have difficulty in getting out of bed/chair with a tendency to fall back.

Occasionally vertebrobasilar territory transient ischemia may be responsible for drop attacks. However, this can be diagnosed only when there are additional transient brainstem symptoms like diplopia, dysarthria or ataxia, immediately following the drop attack.

## NORMAL PRESSURE HYDROCEPHALUS

This is a condition seen in the elderly with a triad of symptoms.
i. Gait disorder: Wide based gait with small steps
ii. Bladder involvement: Urgency and urge incontinence
iii. Memory impairment.

The MR brain shows moderate degree of hydrocephalus (Fig. 14.3) with normal CSF analysis.

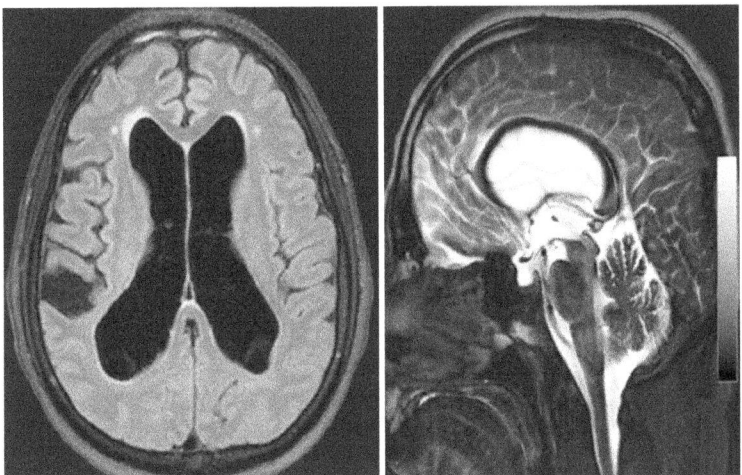

Fig. 14.3: MR brain—normal pressure hydrocephalus.

The symptoms progress over a period of few months. To confirm the diagnosis, the therapeutic test of LP CSF drainage should be done. 30-40 ml of CSF should be drained on alternate days for three sittings. The patient improves first in his gait within 24 to 48 hours. The second symptom to improve is bladder and at times the memory. Subsequently with re-accumulation of CSF the patient's symptoms recur, and LP CSF drainage should be repeated. If the improvement is confirmed a permanent solution like ventriculoperitoneal shunt should be considered.

## FALLS

Falls in elderly is quite common leading to fractures due to frail bones (Tables 14.6 and 14.7).

#### Table 14.6: Common causes of falls.

- Syncope
- Orthostatic hypotension
- Epilepsy
- Myoclonic jerks
- Postural Imbalance
- TIA vertebrobasilar territory
- Sensory neuropathy
- Cognitive impairment
- Visual and auditory impairment
- Gait disorders
- Medications—sedatives

Often even the detailed neurological examination may not give the real cause of frequent falls.

#### Table 14.7: Extrinsic factors for falls in elderly.

- Poor lighting
- Uneven ground
- Ill fitting footwear

### Drop Attacks

Drop attacks are defined as sudden spontaneous falls while standing or walking with preserved consciousness (Table 14.8).

#### Table 14.8: Causes of drop attacks.

- Orthostatic hypotension
- Visual and vestibular disorders
- Gait freezing
- Seizure (Myoclonic jerk, atonic seizure)

Falls with loss of consciouness is a different situation (Table 14.9).

#### Table 14.9: Falls with loss of consciousness—causes.

- Syncope
- Seizure

# CHAPTER 15

# Motor Weakness and Paraplegia

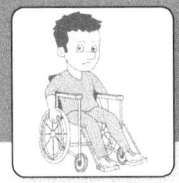

Paraplegia is loss of motor power in both lower limbs; quadriplegia is loss of motor power in all four limbs.

*Motor weakness/paralysis occurs in Table 15.1*:
- Upper motor neuron lesion
- Lower motor neuron lesion
- Neuromuscular junction disorder
- Muscle disease

### Table 15.1: Motor weakness—differential diagnosis.

|  | UMN | LMN | Muscle | Neuromuscular junction |
|---|---|---|---|---|
| Motor Weakness | Distal | Distal/Proximal | Proximal | Fluctuating, fatigability |
| Wasting | Absent | Present/Absent | Absent | Absent |
| Tendon reflexes | Exaggerated | Hypo/Normal | Normal | Normal |
| Plantar | Extensor | Flexor | Flexor | Flexor |
| Associated sensory impairment | +/− Over trunk | +/− Distal | Nil | Nil |
| Bladder involvement | +/− | +/− | − | − |
| Investigations | MR spinal cord | ENMG/MR lumbosacral spine (cauda equina lesion) | CK, EMG | ENMG, Repetitive nerve stimulation; Neostigmine test |
| Common conditions | Acute transverse myelitis | GB syndrome | Acute polymyositis | Generalized myasthenia |

### How to Differentiate Wasting of Muscles—Systemic/Neurogenic Cause?

Generalized wasting of muscles occur due to systemic disorders like malnutrition, cachexia associated with malignancy, tuberculosis. The wasting is *symmetrical* and total loss of *power never occurs*. In neurogenic wasting it is *asymmetric* in distribution with *asymmetric motor weakness*.

## CLINICAL APPROACH TO ACUTE/SUBACUTE PARAPLEGIA

Common causes for paraplegia progressing over 2 to 3 days are listed in Table 15.2.

### Table 15.2: Common causes of acute/subacute UMN paraplegia.
- Demyelinating disorders (MS) (NMO)
- Transverse myelitis
- B12 myelopathy
- Compressive pathology (e.g. abscess, TB)
- Spinal injuries
- Spinal cord infarction

**Case History:** A 36-year-old male presented with fever for 2 days followed by sudden onset of paraplegia and urinary retention. Examination revealed hypotonic areflexic total paraplegia, sensory level at D10 plantar, non-elicitable bladder full.

*Step 1*: *Neurologic deficits*—UMN paraplegia (in view of sensory level and bladder)

*Step 2*: *Anatomical localization*—D10

*Step 3*: *Pathological diagnosis*—Acute onset—inflammatory/demyelination

*Step 4*: *Final diagnosis*—Transverse myelitis/demyelination

Investigation to confirm anatomical localization—MR thoracic spinal cord plain and contrast, swelling of thoracic cord (Fig. 15.1) CSF—inflammatory response.

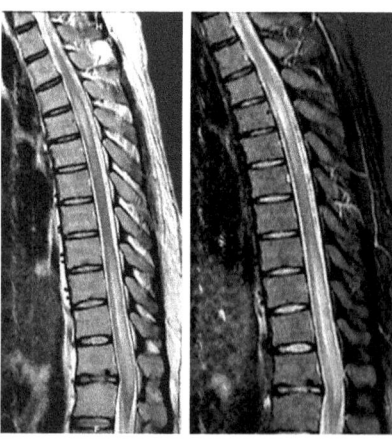

Fig. 15.1: MR thoracic spine—transverse myelitis.

*Diagnosis:* Acute transverse myelitis.

In clinical practice "Transverse Myelitis" (UMN)/GB syndrome (LMN) are commonly encountered.

The management and prognosis is entirely different and so it is imperative to make a proper diagnosis (Table 15.3).

**Table 15.3: Differential features of UMN/LMN lesion in acute paraplegia.**

|  | UMN (e.g. Acute transverse myelitis) | LMN (e.g. GB syndrome) |
|---|---|---|
| Motor system examination |  |  |
| Distribution | Distal > proximal | Proximal > distal |
| Tone | ❏ Hypotonia | Hypotonia |
| Tendon reflexes | ❏ Sluggish/absent | Sluggish/absent |
| Bladder | ❏ Affected (retention) | Unaffected |
| Sensory level | ❏ Present over thorax/abdomen | Absent/distal |

*Case History:* An 18-year-old male was admitted with sudden onset of weakness of left lower limb in the afternoon and required help to walk. The following morning he was unable to get up from bed as he was totally paraplegic. There were no sensory symptoms; bladder was intact. Examination revealed normal tone with no movement at hip and knee, minimal movements at ankle, absent tendon reflexes, plantar flexor. There was minimal sensory impairment over the left lower limb distally.

*Step 1:* Neurological deficit—Flaccid paraplegia, proximal more than distal, distal sensory impairment.

*Step 2:* Anatomical localization—LMN-Radiculoneuropathy. In view of proximal muscle weakness being more pronounced (In UMN distal muscle weakness is more) and distal sensory neuropathy.

*Step 3:* Pathological diagnosis—Acute onset, demyelination.

*Step 4:* Etiological diagnosis—Infective/immune mediated.

*Investigation of choice for anatomical localization:* Nerve conduction studies including F and H reflex.

*Investigation for etiological diagnosis:* CSF examination preferably in 2nd week which shows evidence of inflammatory response—few lymphocytes and increased protein—albuminocytological dissociation and normal sugar.

*Diagnosis:* GB syndrome.

Acute transverse myelitis should be differentiated from demyelinating disorders (MS/NMO) as the management, prognosis differs (Table 15.4).

| Table 15.4: Differential features of transverse myelitis and MS. | | |
|---|---|---|
| Clinical findings | Transverse myelitis | Multiple sclerosis |
| Sensory | ++ | +/– |
| Motor | ++ | ++ |
| Bladder | ++ | +/– |
| MR thoracic cord | Edematous cord with swelling | Demyelinating plaques |
| MR brain | Normal | Demyelinating plaque +/– |
| Past history of similar illness | Nil | +/– |
| CSF inflammatory response | + with more cells | + few cells |
| CSF oligoclonal bands | – | + |
| Management of acute episode | Methylprednisolone | Methylprednisolone/ Plasmapheresis/IgG |
| Disease modifying therapy required | No | Yes |

**Case History:** A 24-year-old female presented with difficulty to walk due to weakness of lower limbs of 3 days duration. Examination showed motor weakness of 3/5 power in all four limbs with brisk reflexes, normal sensations and intact bladder.

*Step 1: Neurological deficit*—UMN quadriparesis, pure motor.
*Step 2: Anatomical localization*—Cervical cord.
*Step 3: Pathological localization*—Acute demyelination/Inflammatory

Investigation for anatomical localization—MR cervical spine which showed demyelinating plaque (Fig. 15.2). CSF—Inflammatory reaction and oligoclonal bands positive.

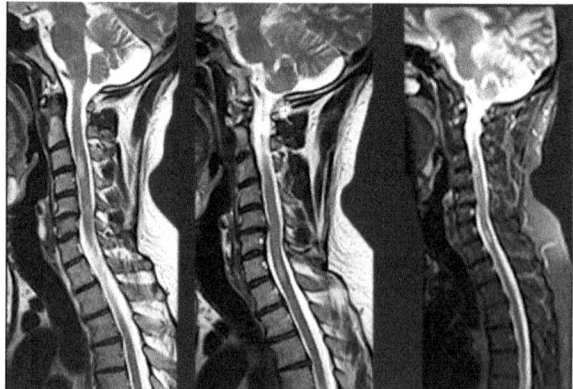

Fig. 15.2: MR cervical spine—demyelinating plaques.

***Diagnosis***: Multiple sclerosis.

MR brain showed demyelinating plaques in the brain which further strengthened the diagnosis of MS (Fig. 15.3).

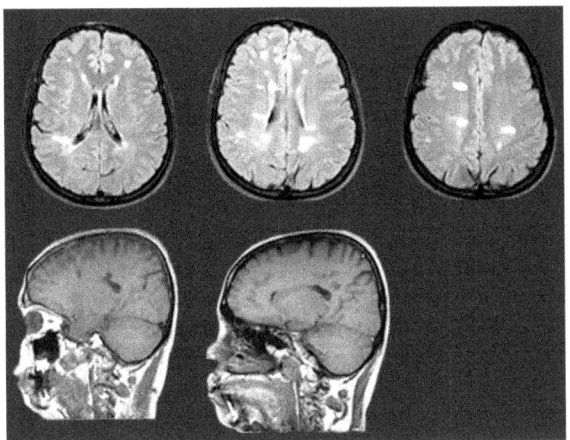

**Fig. 15.3:** MR brain—multiple demyelinating plaques.

### Why should Transverse Myelitis be Differentiated from MS?

In both the conditions the acute management is the same with IV methylprednisolone for 5 days. However, in MS if there is no response, further management consists of plasmapheresis, IV IgG.

Transverse myelitis is one off disease, while MS can relapse, in the same place or involve optic nerves and brainstem. Hence, disease modifying therapy has to be instituted.

### Multiple Sclerosis (MS)

Earlier MS was thought to be rare in India. However with the availability of MR Scans, the identification of MS has increased manifold (Table 15.5).

| Table 15.5: Types of MS. |
|---|
| ❑ Clinically isolated syndrome (CIS) – Any one of the following may be affected optic nerve, spinal cord, brainstem<br>❑ Relapsing remitting MS (RRMS)<br>❑ Secondary progressive MS (SPMS)<br>❑ Primary progressive MS (PPMS)<br>❑ RRMS is the most common. |

As the term multiple sclerosis implies, the demyelinating lesions must be multiple in location and occurring multiple times. The common sites of lesions are optic nerve, spinal cord, brainstem and cerebral hemisphere. The diagnosis is supported by clinical and MR criteria and further evidence with the presence of oligoclonal bands in CSF.

A close associate of this is *Neuromyelitis optica*—demyelination of optic nerves and spinal cord sparing the brain (Fig. 15.4).

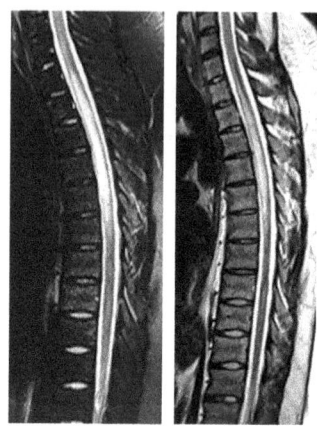

Fig. 15.4: MR cervical spine—long segment demyelination.

## Why should MS be differentiated from NMO?

Though the management of acute episode is similar, the prognosis and disease modifying therapy are totally different (Table 15.6).

| Table 15.6: Differentiating features between MS and NMO. | | |
|---|---|---|
| | MS | NMO |
| Optic nerve | + | + |
| Spinal cord | + Short lesion | + Long lesion > 3 segments (Fig. 15.4) |
| Brain | + | – |
| Symptoms | Less severe | More severe |
| Relapsing remitting | + | + |
| CSF | Oligoclonal bands | – |
| Serum | – | Aquaporin antibodies |
| Treatment of acute episode | Steroids | Steroids |
| Disease modifying therapy | Interferons, glatiramer acetate, natalizumab Dimethyl fumarate Fingolimod Rituximab | Steroids Azathioprine Mycophenolate |

## Management of MS and NMO

*Management of acute episode* of MS and NMO consists of:
a. IV Methylprednisolone 1 gram daily for five days.
b. If the response is poor and neurological disability is significant, the alternative treatments are Plasmapheresis or IV IgG.

## Clinical Approach to Slow Progressive/Chronic UMN Paraplegia

Common Causes of Slow Progressive UMN Paraplegia are Listed in Table 15.7.

| Table 15.7: Common causes of chronic UMN paraplegia. |
| --- |
| ❑ Cervical spondylotic myelopathy |
| ❑ Compressive pathology (e.g. tumor) |
| ❑ Motor neuron disease |
| ❑ Tropical spastic paraplegia (HTLV 1 paraplegia) |
| ❑ Hereditary spastic paraplegia |
| ❑ Fluorosis |
| ❑ Lathyrism |
| ❑ Syphilis |

**Case History:** A 45-year-old male presented with pain in mid back on right side with progressive worsening over two months followed by difficulty in walking due to stiffness of right lower limb. In the third month developed urgency and urge incontinence and frequent falls.

Clinical examination showed a sensory level at D4 in addition to UMN paraparesis.

*Step 1: Neurological deficit*—All three components of paraplegia—UMN paraplegia (spasticity), sensory at D4 and bladder involvement.

*Step 2: Anatomical localization*—In view of sensory level, it is D3.

*Step 3: Pathological diagnosis*—The history is progressive and so the first thought is compressive pathology. The common compressive pathologies are neurofibroma and meningioma both of which are benign tumors and are eminently treatable; TB spine.

**Investigation** for anatomical localization—MR thoracic spine, area of interest D3 level, plain and contrast required for meningioma (vascular tumors), tubercular abscess (inflammatory) (Fig. 15.5).

*Step 4: Etiological diagnosis*—MR thoracic cord showed tubercular abscess compressing the spinal cord. Operated and confirmed histopathologically.

**Diagnosis:** TB spine.

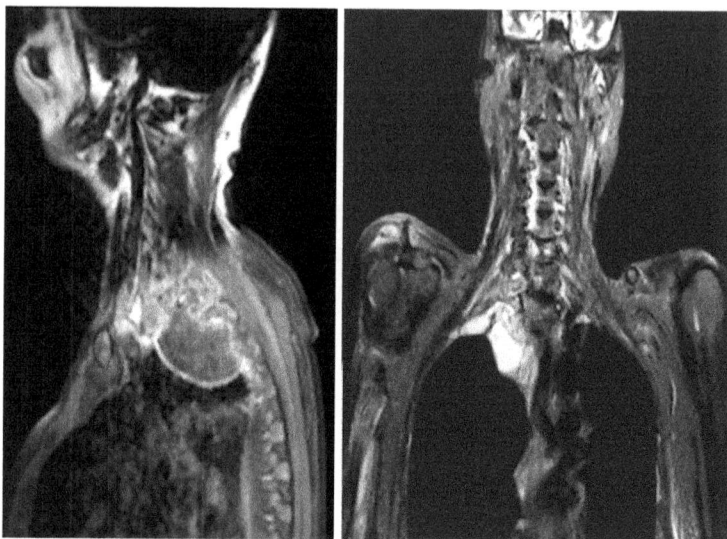

**Fig. 15.5:** MR thoracic spine—D2 tubercular abscess.

Spinal cord compression can be intramedullary (within spinal cord) or extramedullary—intradural or extradural (Table 15.8).

**Table 15.8: Spinal cord lesion—localization.**

| Clinical features | Intramedullary | Extramedullary | |
|---|---|---|---|
| | | Intradural | Extradural |
| Pain | Vague burning pain | Radicular, severe | Bone pain, local, boring |
| Motor paralysis | Bilateral symmetric | Asymmetric | Asymmetric |
| Bladder | Early | Late | Late |
| Sensory | Sacral sparing | Asymmetric early sacral sensory loss | Asymmetric early sacral sensory loss |
| Common causes | Demyelination glioma | Meningioma neurofibroma | Metastasis TB spine |

MR spine differentiates the localization much more precisely (Fig. 15.6).

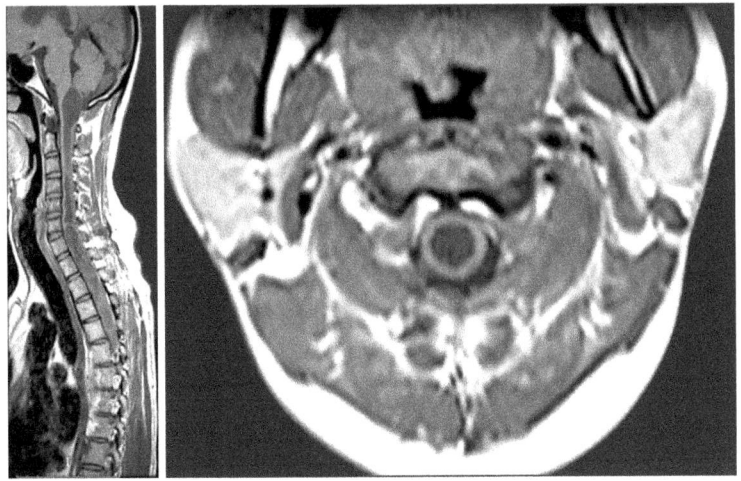

**Fig. 15.6:** MR cervical spine—intramedullary tumors.

***Case History:*** A 65-year-old male diabetic since twenty years complains of progressive difficulty in walking of one and half year duration with tingling and numbness of feet. He was investigated with MR lumbosacral spine which was non-contributory and ENMG confirming peripheral neuropathy. He was told that nothing could be done except controlling the diabetic state. Clinical examination revealed UMN paraparesis with exaggerated reflexes in all four limbs and diminished vibration sense.

*Step 1*: *Neurological deficit*—UMN quadriparesis with posterior column dysfunction.

*Step 2*: *Anatomical localization*—cervical spinal cord.

*Step 3*: *Pathological diagnosis*—slow progressive? benign compression? degenerative.

***Investigation of choice for anatomical localization:*** MR cervical spine, showed compression and constriction of spinal cord at C3,4,5 due to ossification of posterior longitudinal ligament. Surgical decompression was done and the patient improved dramatically. Of course he had peripheral neuropathy due to long standing diabetes, but his difficulty in walking was not due to that.

***Diagnosis:*** Spastic quadriparesis due to cervical cord compression due to ossification of posterior longitudinal ligament (Fig. 15.7).

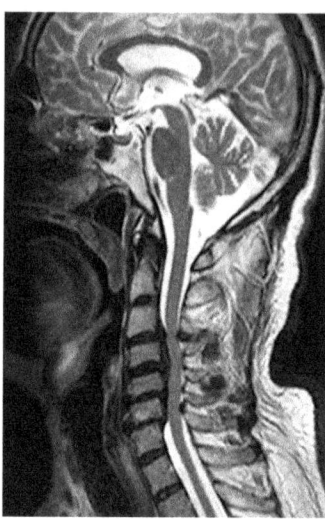

**Fig. 15.7:** MR cervical spine—ossification of posterior longitudinal ligament.

***Message:*** Presence of one disease does not rule out another disease. Clinical examination showed the disability due to spasticity and the spasticity cannot be explained on the basis of peripheral neuropathy.

Always ask yourself what explains the patient's disability, instead of blindly following the investigative results.

***Case History:*** A 65-year-old female presented with difficulty in walking of six months duration and difficulty in talking since three months. She is a known hypertensive and diabetic on appropriate medication. The referring doctor promptly ordered for MR brain (because of speech involvement) and MR entire spine for difficulty in walking! As all these were non-contributory and as the patient had stiffness in limbs with a provisional diagnosis of Parkinson's disease, levodopa was started.

Clinical examination showed wasting of tongue with fasciculations. The other positive findings were spasticity of all four limbs with brisk tendon reflexes and brisk jaw jerk. No sensory deficit and no bladder involvement.

*Step 1*: Neurological deficit—LMN, paralysis of tongue, UMN paralysis (spasticity) of all four limbs with exaggerated reflexes, exaggerated jaw jerk.

*Step 2*: Anatomical localization—UMN bulbar (brisk jaw jerk) and spinal and LMN 12th cranial nerve nucleus in medulla.

*Step 3*: Pathological diagnosis—Slow progressive but with different anatomical localization and pure motor deficits—degenerative disease.

*Step 4*: Final diagnosis—bulbar and spinal motor neuron disease.

*Investigation* of choice to confirm localization—EMG which confirmed evidence of anterior horn cell disease in tongue as well as in hands.

*Diagnosis*: Motor neuron disease.

*Message*: A simple clinical examination would have made a proper diagnosis and avoided unnecessary and expensive investigations.

### Multifocal Motor Neuropathy (MMN)

A rare but treatable disorder often confused for motor neuron disease (Table 15.9).

**Table 15.9: Multifocal motor neuropathy—clinical features.**
- Wasting of small muscles of hand
- Pure motor symptoms, asymmetric, distal, upper limbs > lower limbs
- Fasciculations
- NCV—conduction block
- GM1 antibodies increased
- Treatment—IVIG *steroids worsen the symptoms*

## APPROACH TO CLINICAL DISABILITY DUE TO STIFFNESS OF LIMBS

When the patient's disability is due to stiffness of limbs, the following is the differential diagnosis (Table 15.10).

**Table 15.10: Differential diagnosis of increased muscle tone (stiffness).**

|  | Spasticity | Rigidity | Myotonias | Stiff-person syndrome |
|---|---|---|---|---|
| Increased tone | Antigravity muscles | Both agonists and antagonists | Groups of muscles | Usually paraspinal muscles |
| Tendon reflexes | Exaggerated | Normal/difficult to elicit | Normal | Normal |
| Plantar reflex | Extensor | Flexor | Flexor | Flexor |
| Common causes | Multiple sclerosis MND | Parkinson's disease | Myotonic dystrophy | Stiff person syndrome |

If the patient complains of difficulty to walk due to stiffness of lower limbs it could be spasticity (UMN Lesion), rigidity (extrapyramidal lesion like in Parkinson's disease), occasionally due to myotonia (a muscle disease) or Stiff-person syndrome.

One can visualize the stiff limbs as the patient is walking and the examination will differentiate spasticity (increased tone in antigravity muscles, brisk tendon reflexes, extensor plantar reflex) from rigidity (uniform resistance for both flexors and extensors of the limb).

UMN lesion can manifest as motor weakness or spasticity. If spasticity is the cause of disability medication to reduce spasticity (Baclofen) will improve motor function.

Spasticity as *the cause for disability* (not motor weakness) is observed in few situations e.g. multiple sclerosis, cervical spondylotic myelopathy, motor neuron disease.

Motor weakness *as the cause for disability* in UMN lesion is seen in many other situations like spinal cord compression, transverse myelitis.

***Case History:*** A 48-year-old female presented with history of progressive difficulty in walking due to stiffness and pain in right upper limb of one year duration. MR cervical spine showed C5-6 disc prolapse indenting the cervical cord. She was operated with a diagnosis of cervical spondylotic myelopathy. Her symptoms worsened postoperatively.

Neurological examination showed rigidity of limbs (not spasticity).

***Diagnosis:*** Parkinson's disease.

*There were no tremors.* The pain is due to muscular rigidity.

***Message:*** One should differentiate spasticity from rigidity by basic clinical examination and not be mislead by imaging features.

Infrequently in myotonia (a muscle disorder) severe muscle contraction of the thigh or calf muscles may limit the mobility. Stiff-person syndrome, rarely encountered, causes stiffening of the paraspinal muscles limiting the mobility.

## CLINICAL APPROACH TO SLOW PROGRESSIVE/CHRONIC LMN PARAPLEGIA

***Case History:*** A 45-year-old female presented with low back pain and left lower limb pain of two months duration with difficulty to walk, and to pass urine of one month duration.

*Step 1*: *Neurological deficit*—LMN paraparesis left more than right (hypotonia, areflexia).

Sensory loss in the perianal region, posterior aspect of left thigh L1-S1—left side, S1-S5—right side.

*Step 2*: *Anatomical localization*—Cauda equina lesion.

*Step 3*: *Pathological diagnosis*—Subacute progressive—inflammatory/space occupying lesion.

*Step 4*: *Final diagnosis* depends on investigation.

***Investigation*** for anatomical localization—MR lumbar spine

***Diagnosis:*** Neurofibroma at L1 (Fig. 15.8).

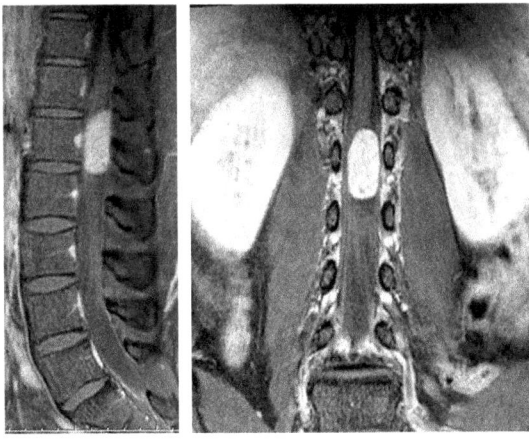

Fig. 15.8: MR lumbar spine neurofibroma.

LMN paralysis is manifested by motor weakness, hypotonia, areflexia. The lesion can be in anterior horn, anterior root, plexus or peripheral nerve (Table 15.11).

Table 15.11: Differential diagnosis of LMN paralysis.

|  | Anterior horn cell | Anterior root | Plexus | Peripheral nerve |
| --- | --- | --- | --- | --- |
| Motor weakness | Proximal/distal | Proximal more than distal | Proximal | Distal |
| Wasting | Prominent | +/– | +/– | +/– |
| Fasciculations | Prominent | +/– | – | – |
| Tendon reflexes | Normal | Hypo/absent | Normal/hypo | Hypo/absent |
| Common causes | Motor neuron disease Poliomyelitis | GB syndrome, Radiculopathy due to disc prolapse (cervical/lumbar) | Plexopathy (Brachial/lumbar) | Diabetes |

***Case History:*** A 56-year-old male non-diabetic, non-hypertensive had acute onset of pain in the lower back, numbness of buttocks and right lower limb, with difficulty to walk, and to pass urine six months ago. All the symptoms cleared the next day without any specific treatment. MR LS spine was unremarkable. The episode repeated two months later and again one month prior to consultation, this time the numbness over buttocks was persisting. Examination revealed decreased pin sensation over the perianal area and posterior aspects of right lower limb and absent right ankle jerk.

### Clinical diagnosis

*Step 1*: *Neurological deficit*—Sensory motor involvement (LMN) of right L5 S1 and bilateral S3,4,5.

*Step 2*: *Anatomical localization*—Lower cauda equina lesion (perianal sensory loss is very significant for localization).

*Step 3*: *Pathological diagnosis*—Three episodes of transient nature— transient ischemia.

*Step 4*: *Etiological diagnosis*—Investigated for spinal AV malformation, confirmed by spinal angiogram and the vessel was embolized. Patient recovered completely over next six weeks.

**Diagnosis:** LMN, paraplegia cauda equina localization due to spinal AV malformation.

**Message:** For episodic LMN lesion consider vascular etiology.

Lesions in lumbar region can manifest as Cauda equina or Conus medullaris disorders (Table 15.12).

Table 15.12: Differential diagnosis of cauda equina—conus medullaris lesion.

|  | Conus medullaris | Cauda equina |
|---|---|---|
| Symptoms | Low back pain +/– | Low back and radicular pain |
| Motor | UMN, LMN combination mild paresis | Pure LMN asymmetric |
| **Reflexes** | | |
| Knee jerk | Present | Absent |
| Ankle jerk | Absent | Absent |
| Plantar | Extensor | Flexor |
| Bulbocavernosus, anal reflex | Absent | Present |
| Sensory | Symmetric perianal (saddle anesthesia) | Asymmetric perianal (saddle anesthesia) |
| Bladder and bowel | Early ++ | Late + |
| Pain | Rare, perineal | Prominent, radicular, asymmetric |

### Finally there are Conversion Disorders Mimicking Paralysis

***Case History:*** A 12-year-old male had an abrupt onset of difficulty in walking preceded by fever for a day. He was diagnosed as GB syndrome/transverse myelitis and appropriately investigated with MR spine, nerve conduction studies and CSF all of which were normal. On the third day of illness he develop jerky movements of hands and head, memory lapse—not being able to recognize school mates and teachers. MR brain and EEG were normal. A clinical diagnosis of ADEM (acute demyelinating encephalomyelitis) was considered and he was administered IV methylprednisolone for five days with no improvement. He continued to be in the same state and was transferred to this hospital after four weeks. Neurological examination revealed normal power in the lower limbs when examined on the couch. However, when made to walk he had difficulty and was walking on the lateral surface of the feet (both sides). This is something very unusual and raised a suspicion of conversion disorder (psychological problem). Further history revealed that the boy who was studying in Bengaluru was shifted to a school in Kanpur four months ago (as the parents were transferred there) and his memory was affected selectively for his classmates and teachers!! All treatment was stopped and he was referred to psychiatry for counseling. His parents assured him that he would not be sent back to Kanpur. He recovered completely in the following three to four weeks.

***Diagnosis:*** Conversion disorder.

## QUADRIPLEGIA

All causes and features of paraplegia and quadriplegia are the same except for localization to cervical cord.

## MYOPATHY

Motor weakness due to muscle disorders (myopathy) are discussed in Chapter 17)

## MYASTHENIA

Diseases due to neuromuscular disorder (myasthenia) is characterized by fluctuating motor weakness, fatigability, usually starts with diplopia ptosis.

Whenever a patient complains of tiredness, one is likely to dismiss it as a non-specific symptom. However, if the history suggests *disabling motor weakness* relieved by *brief rest*, one should consider myasthenia. For example, if the person becomes so tired after climbing a few steps that he is unable to stand, but after resting for a few minutes, he resumes climbing, then think of myasthenia, which can be confirmed by therapeutic test/EMG.

When there are symptoms like fluctuating ptosis or diplopia, then it is easy to diagnose. But do not miss when it affects only the lower limbs, because it is eminently treatable. There is no use of investigating B12, Vitamin D levels and pumping them into the patient! Disabling *fatigability is the key word*.

**Case History:** A 56-year-old female diabetic and hypertensive presented with history of difficulty in talking, eating food and nasal regurgitation of one week duration. Obviously the immediate diagnosis is brainstem stroke, particularly in view of the age and background history of hypertension and diabetes. MR brain was normal.

The point to note is that in spite of cranial nerves (7, 9, 10) being affected, there were no symptoms or signs of long tract (corticospinal, cerebellar) involvement! A point against brainstem stroke.

*Step 1: Neurological deficit*—Multiple lower cranial nerve palsy.

*Step 2: Anatomical localization*—In nerves as they are coursing at the base of brain. Not in brainstem as there were no long tract signs like UMN, cerebellar etc.

*Step 3: Pathological diagnosis*—Further history revealed that *symptoms were fluctuating* within a day itself, pointing to a diagnosis of bulbar myasthenia, which was confirmed by EMG and therapeutic test with neostigmine.

***Diagnosis:*** Bulbar myasthenia.

***Message:*** More detailed history is important when bulbar symptoms are isolated without hemiparesis or ataxia. It is also important to note that this patient did not have the classical onset of myasthenia with ptosis and diplopia (Table 15.13). If there is no history of fluctuating symptoms, then polyneuritis cranialis to be considered.

**Table 15.13: Clinical features of myasthenia.**

- Clinical—Fatigability is the benchmark for the diagnosis
    - Episodic weakness, diplopia, ptosis
    - Bulbar—dysphagia, dysphonia
- EMG—Repetitive nerve stimulation—Fatigue response
- Serum—AChR antibody increased
- Therapeutic response—To neostigmine im/iv
- Management—Steroids, pyridostigmine, mycophenolate
    - Azathioprine
- Thymectomy—in selected cases
- Myasthenic crisis—Plasmapheresis, IV IgG

**Table 15.14: Episodic weakness: causes.**

- Hypokalemia, hyperkalemia
- Hypercalcemia
- Hypermagnesemia
- Hypophosphatemia
- Myasthenia

**Table 15.15: Muscle weakness with cramps: causes.**

- MND
- Radiculopathy
- Neuropathy

The main features of episodic enduring motor weakness (not fluctuating motor weakness) and cramps associated with muscle weakness are described in Tables 15.14 and 15.15.

# CHAPTER 16

# Neurogenic Bladder

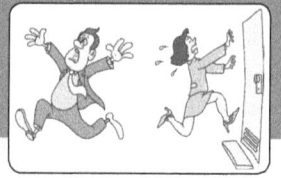

Neurology is perceived as a difficult branch of medicine and the bladder as the most difficult subject to understand!

The bladder is a very simple organ with simple functions. The anatomical structures are detrusor, internal or smooth muscle sphincter, which is an involuntary muscle, and external or striated muscle sphincter which is under voluntarily control. The function of the bladder is storage of urine and periodically empty it.

The dominant innervation is from the parasympathetic nervous system derived from the intermediolateral column of sacral cord (S2,3,4). The sympathetic innervation is from the intermediolateral column of thoraco-lumbar cord (D10-L2). The voluntary external sphincter is innervated by the pudendal nerve derived from the S2-4 anterior horn cells.

The main center is in the pontomesencephalic reticular formation (pons and medulla).

Voluntary control of bladder is on the medial surface of the frontal lobe. Up to a point, the voluntary control through striated external sphincter can be executed to initiate or stop micturition.

The neurogenic bladder is of two types: UMN, LMN. One can understand the neurogenic bladder better when it is compared to the UMN, LMN lesions of paraparesis.

There are several classifications of neurogenic bladder, the simplest and most practical is given in Table 16.1.

### Table 16.1: Classification of neurogenic bladders.

a. Hypertonic hyperreflexic bladder (UMN lesion)
- *Hyperreflexic bladder (UMN) with coordinated sphincters*
- *Hyperreflexic bladder (UMN) without coordination of sphincters*

b. Hypotonic hyporeflexic bladder (LMN lesion)
- *Hyporeflexic bladder (LMN) with coordinated sphincters*
- *Hyporeflexic bladder (LMN) without coordination of sphincters*

## SYMPTOMS OF BLADDER DYSFUNCTION

- ❑ Frequency, urgency, urge incontinence (UMN).
- ❑ Hesitancy/difficulty to pass urine, overflow incontinence (LMN).

Common causes of bladder symptoms are largely due to non-neurological causes (Table 16.2).

### Table 16.2: Common cause of frequency, urgency.
- Anxiety
- Cystitis
- Bladder stone
- Neurogenic cause for frequency is infrequent and is accompanied by other neurologic features—paraparesis, altered reflexes

*Stand alone neurogenic bladder*, i.e. *isolated bladder symptoms due to neurological cause, is very rare.*

### Hyperreflexic Bladder (UMN Lesion)

In UMN lesion, the limb muscles are spastic with exaggerated reflexes. The same applies to bladder which is hyperreflexic and contracts at a smaller volume. This results in frequent emptying of the bladder, *(frequency)*. Later on, the bladder contraction is so fast that there is no time to reach the bathroom causing *urgency* to pass urine which at times results in *urge incontinence.*

Normally, when the bladder contracts the internal sphincter spontaneously relaxes to facilitate emptying of the bladder. However, in some types of UMN lesions the internal sphincter does not coordinate with the bladder contraction thus resulting in residual urine *in spite* of frequency and urgency. The residual urine, which if not detected, may lead to back pressure effects and renal failure. *Hence, in every UMN bladder, even though the patient says he is passing urine frequently and adequately one should do an ultrasound for postvoid residual urinary volume.*

*Hyperreflexic bladder (UMN) with coordinated sphincters*: When the bladder contracts, the internal sphincter opens up, thus facilitating the emptying of the bladder. This is seen in early lesions of UMN as in multiple sclerosis, frontal lobe lesions and dementia.

Abdominal ultrasound for postvoid residual urine will be less than 50 ml.

*Hyper reflexic bladder (UMN) without coordination of sphincters*: When the bladder contracts, the internal sphincter does not completely open up resulting in partial emptying of the bladder. There will be *significant post-void residual urine* in the bladder. This is seen in advanced stages of multiple sclerosis.

**Case History:** A 26-year-old female presented with the primary symptom of frequency and urge incontinence of one week duration. Examination revealed mild spasticity of lower limbs with exaggerated tendon reflexes.

Her bladder symptoms were identified as due to neurological cause. MR thoracic spine showed demyelinating plaque.

**Diagnosis:** Multiple sclerosis.

In intrinsic cord lesions, early bladder involvement occurs, which means that the patient's mobility is near normal but is disturbed by neurogenic (UMN) bladder. In contrast, in extrinsic spinal cord compression, motor weakness is predominant with bladder symptoms appearing much later by which time there is considerable locomotor disability (for more details on paraplegia, *see* Chapter 15).

The symptomatic management of frequency, urgency is by using anticholinergic drugs (Table 16.3).

**Table 16.3: Anticholinergic drugs in hyperreflexic bladder.**
- Oxybutynin (Ditropan XL, Oxytrol)
- Tolterodine (Terol)
- Darifenacin (Darif)
- Solifenacin (Soliten)

In men with urge incontinence, due to prostate hyperplasia, alpha-blockers (Table 16.4) are used which relax bladder neck muscles and muscle fibers in the prostate and make it easier to empty the bladder.

**Table 16.4: Alpha blockers.**
- Tamsulosin (Urimax)
- Alfuzosin (Flotral)
- Silodosin (Silodal)
- Terazosin (Hytrin)
- Prazosin (Minipress)
- Doxazosin (Doxacard)

### Hypotonic Hyporeflexic Bladder (LMN Lesion)

LMN lesion of the limb muscles results in hypotonia and hyporeflexia. The bladder too is hypotonic and hyporeflexic with early symptoms of hesitancy and difficulty to pass urine as the bladder is not contracting properly. Later retention and overflow incontinence occurs. The postvoid residual urine will give us a clue to the severity of the condition.

**Management** consists of mechanical compression of the bladder from above downwards over the lower abdomen (Credés method) to facilitate bladder evacuation. In addition, cholinergic drugs (urecholine) to stimulate bladder contraction is used. This method is unlikely to succeed over a long period of time or in advanced lesions at which time clean intermittent self-catheterization (CISC) is advocated.

The type of neurogenic bladder (UMN/LMN) is recognized by accompanying UMN/LMN clinical features (Table 16.5).

### Table 16.5: Differentiating of UMN, LMN bladder.

| | UMN | LMN |
|---|---|---|
| Symptoms | Urgency, frequency, urge incontinence | Hesitancy, difficulty to pass urine, Retention, overflow incontinence |
| Signs | Bladder normal | Distended |
| Muscle tone lower limbs | Spastic | Hypotonic |
| Tendon reflexes | Exaggerated | Sluggish/absent |
| Plantar | Extensor | Flexor |
| Lesion | Spinal cord | Cauda equina |
| Common causes | Thoracic cord lesion—MS, tumors | Cauda equina tumors autonomic neuropathy |

*Case History:* A 26-year-old male presented with progressive difficulty in passing urine over the previous six weeks and was also unable to appreciate the fullness of bladder. Three months earlier he had a fall from a height of six feet, landing on his buttocks. However, he was able to get up immediately, had a little low backache but was normally ambulant. His lumbar spine X-rays showed compression fracture at L1 vertebra. Neurological examination showed that both his lower limbs were totally normal with no sensory involvement. A specific sensory examination over perianal area revealed total loss of touch and pain, thus confirming neurogenic LMN bladder.

### Message

LMN neurogenic bladder is confirmed by sensory loss *over perianal region (Same segments—S2,3,4—for bladder and perianal sensations).* Routine motor and sensory system examination was normal.

### Clean Intermittent Self-catheterization (CISC)

CISC is indicated in both UMN and LMN bladder whenever postvoid residual urine is more than 50-100 ml. If the residual urine builds up it can cause back pressure effects resulting in hydronephrosis and eventually renal failure. The patient is trained to catheterize himself or herself four times a day. The catheter need not be sterilized, nor there is a need for disposable catheter. The catheter should be washed with soap and water under the tap, after use, allowed to dry and then placed in a plastic pouch and should be carried in the pocket. Many patients after traumatic spinal cord injury, multiple sclerosis, who become ambulant with residual urinary symptoms are greatly helped by CISC.

### Urinary Incontinence

Urinary Incontinence is defined as "Involuntary loss of urine, objectively demonstrable and is a social and hygienic problem" (Table 16.6).

**Table 16.6: Types of incontinence.**

a. Urge incontinence
 - Myogenic (detrusor instability)
 - Neurogenic (detrusor hyperreflexia—UMN lesion)
b. Overflow incontinence (LMN Lesion)
c. Genuine stress incontinence
 - *Involuntary loss of urine due to raised intra abdominal pressure.* Detrusor unaffected.

***Genuine stress incontinence (GSI)***—is manifested by leakage of urine due to increased abdominal pressure, e.g. sneezing, coughing, straining or even a hearty laugh!! This happens due to pelvic floor weakness in women as a result of deliveries/pelvic surgery and in men following prostatic surgery. It is commonly seen in 10-15% of women aged above 40 years.

The treatment consists of strengthening the pelvic floor by Kegel exercises, sometimes aided by vaginal cones. The pharmacological treatment consists of adrenergic agonists—pseudoephedrine, imipramine, ephedrine, HRT.

It is important to differentiate urge incontinence (Neurological) from Genuine stress incontinence (non-neurological) (Table 16.7).

**Table 16.7: Differentiating features of urge incontinence and genuine stress incontinence.**

| | Urge incontinence (neurogenic) | Genuine stress incontinence (non-neurologic) |
|---|---|---|
| Symptoms | Urgency, frequency, urge incontinence | ❑ Stress incontinence<br>❑ Previous history of vaginal delivery, pelvic floor surgery |
| Signs | Of UMN paresis (hypertonia, hyper reflexia) | ❑ Nil |
| Abdomen ultrasound for bladder | Pre void—small quantity<br>Post void—normal/residual urine | ❑ Normal<br>❑ Normal |
| Management | Anticholinergics | ❑ Pelvic floor exercises |

*Nocturnal enuresis* can be primary where there has been no bladder control since birth or secondary where the bladder control was established but was lost again, causing enuresis. Commonly the primary variety is seen. Normally by age 5, bladder control is established. However, particularly in boys, it may sometimes take even up to 10 years. The treatment consists of Wet-alarm, imipramine, desmopressin nasal spray, (ADH analog of post-pituitary hormone, which causes reduced nocturnal urine production; Hyponatremia, is a side-effect).

***Case history of a 45-year-old female:*** This is an interesting case of frequency, urgency and at times urge incontinence. This lady, a high profile executive, consulted several specialists—neurologists and urologists, for symptoms of frequency, urgency and urge incontinence. It was so bad that she had to use incontinence pads during board meetings and was always on the lookout for a rest room whenever she went out. All investigations were normal. Finally, basics were looked into. She was asked to keep a chart of the intake of all fluids including water and the number of times she had to use the rest room and the quantity of urine. A week later when the chart was reviewed, it was found that the intake of water itself was 3-4 liters per day. On questioning she informed that a naturopath had told her that she should drink that much water to maintain good health! The treatment was simply to restrict fluid intake to normal quantity!

# CHAPTER 17

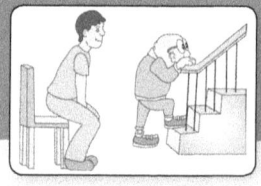

# Difficulty to Get up from Squatting/Climbing Stairs

### Doctor I have Difficulty to Get up from Squatting Position/Indian Toilet Seat

The characteristic features of proximal muscle weakness is *difficulty to get up from squatting position/Indian toilet, difficulty to climb stairs*, but once on their feet a person can walk without much problem, can wear and grip slippers normally (distal muscles normal). This discrepancy in muscle weakness *is diagnostic of proximal muscle weakness*. This should be differentiated from a person who has difficulty in getting up from squatting, *as well as* difficulty to walk, wear slippers, etc. which occurs under several circumstances like Parkinson's disease, upper motor neuron (UMN) and lower motor neuron (LMN) paraparesis.

The proximal muscle weakness is due to neurogenic causes (commonly motor root but also anterior horn cell, plexus) or myogenic (muscle diseases).

There are four parameters to differentiate neurogenic from myogenic cause. They are: clinical, biochemical [creatine kinase (CK)], electrophysiological (ENMG) and finally muscle biopsy (Table 17.1). All the four parameters do not concur and when they are at variance with each other it is the clinical judgment which rules the roost. This is because muscle biopsy tissue may not be representative of the underlying disease due to wrong choice of muscle, i.e. biopsied muscle when minimally affected or maximally affected with burnt out stage does not yield the proper information. Biopsy should be done in a muscle which is actively involved. Similarly in ENMG the sampled muscle and nerve may not be representative of the illness. The CK level when raised greatly is suggestive of not only a muscle disease but an *active muscle disease*. If the CK is done when the disease is quiescent, obviously levels will be normal. Considering these variations in the investigation it is the clinical judgment which is the ultimate deciding factor.

## Table 17.1: Differential features of proximal muscle weakness.

| | Neurogenic | Myogenic |
|---|---|---|
| History | Tingling, numbness, paresthesia, radicular pain | Muscle pain, cramp |
| | *Neurogenic* | *Myogenic* |
| Motor system | ❑ Proximal muscle weakness<br>❑ Normal/wasting<br>❑ Hypotonia/fasciculations | ❑ Proximal muscle weakness<br>❑ Normal/hypertrophy of muscles<br>❑ Normal/hypotonia |
| Tendon reflexes | Absent | Present |
| Sensory | Impaired | Normal |
| Biochemical - CK | Normal | Elevated |
| Electrophysiology ENMG | Neurogenic | Myogenic |
| Histopathology muscle biopsy | Neurogenic atrophy (group atrophy) | Myogenic (varying size and shape of muscle fibers) |
| Common causes | ❑ Radiculopathy—GBS, CIDP<br>❑ Anterior horn cell disease<br>❑ Plexopathy | Polymyositis, muscular dystrophy |

## I. NEUROGENIC PROXIMAL MUSCLE WEAKNESS

Neurogenic causes can be at different anatomical sites (Table 17.2).

### Table 17.2: Neurogenic causes—localization.

❑ Anterior horn cell—Motor neuron disease
❑ Motor root—acute – GB syndrome (AIDP)
　　　　　　　chronic—(CIDP)
❑ Plexus—brachial plexopathy
　　　　　lumbar plexopathy

**Case History:** A 25-year-old male presented with fever for three days, followed by tingling and numbness of feet and difficulty to get up from squatting. Examination showed proximal muscle weakness in lower limbs, absent tendon reflexes, distal sensory impairment over feet; bladder was unaffected.

*Step 1: Neurologic deficit*—LMN paraparesis (hypotonia, absent tendon reflexes).
　　　Distal sensory impairment over feet.

*Step 2*: *Anatomical localization*—Motor roots and peripheral sensory nerve
*Step 3*: *Pathologic diagnosis*—In view of short history—demyelination
*Step 4*: *Etiological diagnosis*—Post-febrile radiculoneuropathy—GB syndrome/ AIDP.

*Investigation for confirming anatomical localization*—Nerve conduction velocity (NCV) including F waves.

***Final diagnosis*:** *GB syndrome (AIDP)*
GB syndrome is a common cause for acute/subacute LMN paralysis.

***Case History*:** A 45-year-old male presented with low back pain of 15 days, three days later he developed difficulty to walk. MR LS spine showed L5-S1 disc prolapse, advised surgery. Examination showed bilateral ankle dorsi and plantar flexor 0/5 power, knee flexor 2/5, hip 3/5 abductors, bilateral ankle reflex absent, knee reflex just elicitable. Sensory normal.

*Step 1*: *Neurological deficit*—Pure LMN paralysis affecting hip, knee and ankle.

*Step 2*: *Anatomical localization*—L2, 3, 4, 5 S1 roots, L4-5 disc prolapse in MR scan is not relevant as at this level the hip and the knee (L2,3) will not be affected!

*Step 3*: *Pathological diagnosis*—Demyelinating radiculopathy.

The diagnosis is GB syndrome and confirmed by the nerve conduction studies and F response. Patient improved remarkably with IV, IgG.

***Diagnosis*:** GB syndrome.

***Message*:** Always have a clinical diagnosis, with firm anatomical localization, that way one will not be mislead by investigations (here MR showed lesion at L 5-S1 while clinical localization is at L2, 3).

The diagnosis of GB syndrome in the first few days is entirely on clinical grounds as the nerve conduction may be totally normal in early stages. At the same time immediate starting of the treatment is necessary to prevent worsening of symptoms. Clinical diagnosis is established by rapidly progressive *pure LMN motor paraplegia* or quadriplegia with bladder being unaffected and at times associated with distal sensory neuropathy. The clue for the diagnosis is involvement of the neck flexors and LMN facial palsy, when it is present, both of which conclusively rule out spinal cord involvement. The differential diagnosis is often between GB syndrome and transverse myelitis. In the latter there is sensory level and bladder involvement.

(For further information *see* Chapter 15).

## MANAGEMENT OF GB SYNDROME

The most common cause is immune mediated disorder, the treatment is to address this issue. In earlier days steroids were the main stay of treatment but recently the choice is between IV immunoglobulin (IgG) 400 mg/kg/day (20-30 gm per day) for 5 consecutive days or plasmapheresis on alternate days for 5 sittings. IgG is decidedly very expensive (₹4-5 lakhs for one course) but easy to administer, while plasmapheresis is relatively cheaper (1-2 lakhs for the course) but is cumbersome and can be done only where hemodialysis facilities are available. As many of our patients cannot afford either of them, IV methylprednisolone 1 gm in 100 mL saline at the rate of 30 drops per minute for 5 days is administered.

Generally the disease progress rapidly over 8-12 days then stabilizes and starts improving at which time physiotherapy is the main stay of the treatment.

The indication for treatment is when the disease is still progressive, threatening respiratory involvement which is the main cause for mortality. However if the patient is seen two weeks after the onset of illness, when the disease is already stabilized or patient is already spontaneously improving then there is no need to institute the expensive therapy!

***Case History:*** A 45-year-old female presented with slow progressive difficulty in getting up from Indian toilet seat, which gradually increased to difficulty in climbing stairs and also difficulty to comb hair and keep kitchen articles on to the upper shelves. The duration of the illness was about 6 months. On probing there were distal sensory symptoms like tingling and numbness. Examination revealed proximal muscle weakness, more in the lower limbs than upper limbs with absent tendon reflexes and normal sensation.

*Step 1: The neurological deficits*—Proximal muscle weakness, LMN.

*Step 2: Anatomical localization*—Anterior root (motor radiculopathy) with sensory neuropathy.

*Step 3: Pathological diagnosis*—Slow progressive, may be demyelinative. The radiculopathies can be acute in nature (GB syndrome), sub acute or chronic CIDP. This case illustrates CIDP—an eminently treatable condition which should be recognized early and *not be confused with untreatable myopathies.*

*Investigation to confirm the anatomical localization* is nerve conduction studies—F and H responses. The other investigation that suggests the inflammatory nature of motor roots is the CSF showing raised protein with normal sugar and very few lymphocytes.

IV methylprednisolone 1 gram daily in 100 ml saline at the rate of 30 drops per minute for 5 days remarkably improved the motor power and this treatment may have to be repeated when it relapses.

***Diagnosis:*** CIDP (chronic immune mediated demyelinating polyneuropathy).

***Case History:*** A 65-year-old male presented with tingling paresthesia of feet, difficulty in getting up from squatting position and slow walking of three months duration. He is a known diabetic with ischemic heart disease and is on regular treatment.

## Clinical Diagnosis

a. *Neurological deficit*: Proximal muscle weakness with absent knee and ankle reflexes (LMN) and distal sensory impairment in the feet
b. *Anatomical localization*: Radiculoneuropathy
c. *Pathological diagnosis*: Demyelinating disease
d. *Etiological diagnosis*: Diabetic.

*Investigation for confirming anatomical localization*—nerve conduction velocity (NCV).

Patient was earlier investigated with MR brain, which showed multiple lacunar infarcts which was followed by carotid Doppler which showed 80% stenosis of both internal carotid artery and hence the referral. With the clinical diagnosis of diabetic radiculoneuropathy these investigations have no clinical relevance. Nerve conduction study confirmed the diagnosis.

**Final Diagnosis:** *Diabetic radiculoneuropathy.*

**Message:** Clinical diagnosis is supreme, do not depend on incidental abnormalities in randomly done investigations!!

## MANAGEMENT

Diabetic radiculopathy/plexopathy is partially immune-mediated and responds well to IV methylprednisolone 1 gm daily × 5 days. The temporary increase in glucose should be managed by insulin. If steroids fail, IV IgG should be administered. Usually patients respond well to these therapies and can walk independently. Of course the underlying diabetic state should be controlled well to prevent recurrence.

**Case History:** A 25-year-old male laborer complained of difficulty in lifting heavy gunny bags from the floor to the table, of two years duration, which initially was not bothering him much but subsequently reduced his efficiency so much so that he was on the verge of losing the job. He had no symptoms referable to distal muscles in upper limb, cranial nerves or lower limbs. He also volunteered the information that there was wasting and twitching of the muscles of the shoulder girdle. From the history, the diagnosis is proximal muscle weakness in the upper limbs and whenever the *proximal muscle weakness starts in the upper limbs* or is confined to the upper limbs it is always a neurological cause (could be neurogenic or myogenic) and effectively rules out systemic causes. Additionally this patient had wasting of muscles and fasciculation which immediately confirms the neurogenic origin of the proximal muscle weakness.

*Step 1*: *Neurological deficits*—Proximal muscle weakness in upper limbs—neurogenic; in view of atrophy, fasciculations.

*Step 2*: *Anatomical localization* could be anterior horn, anterior root or brachial plexus. In view of wasting and fasciculation and pure motor signs the likely localization is anterior horn cells. Motor radiculopathy (like CIDP) is a possibility, however the wasting and fasciculation starting in the upper limbs is untenable. Brachial plexopathy is ruled out as it is a *mixture of motor and sensory symptoms and signs.*

*Step 3*: *Pathological diagnosis*—Slow progressive anterior horn cell disease. Any neurological illness which is relentlessly progressive for more than a year or two is mostly degenerative. Hence we have a degenerative disease affecting the anterior horn cells in cervical cord bilaterally.

*Step 4*: *Etiological diagnosis* is motor neuron disease slotted into spinal muscular atrophy.

*The investigation of choice to confirm the anatomical localization* is electromyography (EMG) which confirmed the diagnosis.

**Diagnosis:** Spinal muscular atrophy.

**Case History:** A 35-year-old male after a brief febrile illness developed pain, paresthesia over right shoulder, which disappeared after a few days. This was followed by difficulty in doing activities like combing hair, washing the head, brushing teeth which shows that it is proximal muscle weakness. Examination revealed right shoulder girdle weakness, with a small coin size area of hypoesthesia at the site of deltoid insertion.

**Diagnosis:** Right brachial plexopathy (brachial neuritis).

**Case History:** An 18-year-old male previously a very healthy individual woke up one morning and noticed difficulty in walking and was rushed to the hospital. Examination revealed bilateral foot drop with absent ankle reflex and normal sensory. In addition there was difficulty to get up from squatting which shows that it is proximal muscle weakness.

a. *Neurological deficit*: Bilateral foot drop with proximal muscle weakness.
b. *Anatomical localization*: Neurogenic—absent tendon reflexes, bilateral symmetrical, possibility of radiculopathy.
c. *Pathological diagnosis,* acute onset—Inflammatory (demyelination) or metabolic (hypokalemia), serum potassium was very low (2.5 mEq/l) with corresponding changes in the ECG.

*Correction of potassium resulted in total recovery by next morning.*

**Diagnosis:** Hypokalemic paralysis; resulting in inexcitability of muscle membrane.

**Message:** In *abrupt onset* of disabling motor paresis *after waking up from sleep* one should suspect hypokalemic paralysis which is eminently treatable. Further history revealed he had a sumptuous dinner the previous night at a marriage party! Hypokalemic paralysis is precipitated by a high carbohydrate meal.

## MYOGENIC PROXIMAL MUSCLE WEAKNESS

Myogenic proximal muscle weakness occurs due to several systemic causes which are eminently treatable. Not all muscle diseases are due to neurological problems (Table 17.3).

Table 17.3: Differential diagnosis of proximal muscle weakness of myogenic origin.

|  | Systemic causes | Neurological causes |
|---|---|---|
| Proximal Muscle Weakness | | |
| Lower limbs | + | + |
| Upper limbs | – | + |
| CK | Normal/mildly elevated | Moderate to severely elevated |
| EMG | Normal/mildly abnormal | Abnormal |
| Histopathology | Normal/nonspecific | Abnormal |
| Common causes | Vit D, Vit B12 deficiency, endocrine dysfunction, e.g. hypothyroid | Polymyositis, muscular dystrophy |

The differential diagnosis when proximal muscle weakness is seen only in the lower limbs is systemic causes *and* neurologic causes. When it affects upper limbs also or starts in the upper limbs *it is always due to a neurological cause*. Common myogenic causes are mentioned in Table 17.4.

Table 17.4: Common causes of myogenic proximal muscle weakness.

**Systemic causes**
- Metabolic—Diabetes
- Endocrinal—Hypothyroidism, hyperthyroidism
  —Addison's disease, hyperparathyroidism
- Deficiency—Vit B12, Vit D
- Medication—Statins, steroids
- Toxic—Alcohol

**Neurological causes**
- Polymyositis—Viral, immune-mediated
- Muscular dystrophy
- Paraneoplastic myopathy

It is mandatory to investigate for a treatable disorder in all myopathies by doing a metabolic, endocrinal and nutritional work up which include T3, FT4, TSH, Vitamin B12 and Vitamin D levels, serum calcium, phosphorus, alkaline phosphatase and CK, and appropriate endocrine work up.

**Case History:** A 50-year-old female complained of insidious onset of progressive difficulty in walking over a few months and required more and more help initially to get up from Indian toilet seat, and subsequently requiring support to get up from a chair also. She also had difficulty to climb the staircase. The examination showed proximal muscle weakness in the lower limb 2/5 power with distal muscles 5/5 power. The *knee reflex was brisk* and she also complained of pain in the thigh muscles. There were no sensory or bladder deficits.

*Step 1*: *Neurological deficit* proximal muscle weakness only in lower limbs.
*Step 2*: *Anatomical localization*—Myogenic (muscle disease). Pain in thigh muscles and absence of sensory symptoms and signs favor myogenic.
*Step 3*: *Pathological diagnosis*—Painful proximal muscle weakness extending over a period of several months and slowly progressive can be an inflammatory disease, e.g. polymyositis. This patient had *painful proximal muscle weakness with brisk reflexes* suggestive of Vitamin D deficiency myopathy. This clinical combination is seen almost exclusively in Vitamin D deficiency. In polymyositis, reflexes are normal and CK is raised.

*Investigation for anatomical localization*—CK and EMG was normal
*Step 4*: *Etiological diagnosis* is by estimation of serum Vit D, calcium. Both were low with elevated alkaline phosphatase. After taking Vit D for a couple of months, patient started walking unaided.

**Diagnosis:** Vit D deficiency myopathy.

**Message:** Painful proximal muscle weakness with brisk tendon reflexes is due to Vit D deficiency—an eminently treatable condition (Table 17.5).

### Table 17.5: Clinical features of Vitamin D deficiency myopathy.

- Proximal muscle weakness in lower limbs only
- Pain in pelvic bones (may be mistaken as "painful proximal muscle weakness")
- Brisk knee reflexes (Due to hypocalcemia)
- Pelvic squeeze elicits pain
- CK, EMG, muscle biopsy—Normal/marginally abnormal
- Low Vit D and calcium
- Remarkable recovery with Vit D and calcium supplement

Inflammatory myopathies are a distinct group of muscle disorders (Table 17.6).

### Table 17.6: Inflammatory myopathies.

| | |
|---|---|
| **Clinical features** | <ul><li>Painful symmetric proximal muscle weakness</li><li>Initially lower limbs, later upper limbs</li><li>Tendon reflexes—normal/hypo</li></ul> |
| **Investigations** | <ul><li>CK—moderate to high elevated</li><li>EMG—Myopathic pattern</li><li>Muscle biopsy—inflammatory changes</li></ul> |
| **Common causes** | <ul><li>Viral polymyositis</li><li>Polymyositis (immune-mediated)</li><li>Dermatomyositis</li></ul> |

While muscle disorders are characterized by weakness as a principle symptom associated pain is a feature of a few conditions (Table 17.7).

### Table 17.7: Muscle disease with pain—causes.
- Polymyositis (viral, immune-mediated)
- Statin induced myopathy
- Hypothyroid myopathy

**Case History:** A 30-year-old male farm laborer had irregular high fever for 5 days followed by severe pain in the thigh muscles and difficulty to stand or walk even with support. There was no history of tingling or numbness, was not a known diabetic or hypertensive. The clinical diagnosis is painful proximal muscle weakness on a background of febrile illness—polymyositis. Neurological examination showed muscle tenderness of quadriceps and calf muscles proximal muscle weakness (after a dose of anti-inflammatory medication the pain considerably reduced but there was proximal weakness of iliopsoas and quadriceps). So the disability here was both due to pain as well as muscle weakness. Reflexes were normal, there were no sensory changes and the distal muscles power was 5/5.

*Step 1: Neurological deficit*—Painful, tender proximal muscle weakness in the lower limbs of a very short duration (unlike painful proximal muscle weakness of several months duration in case of vitamin D deficiency myopathy).

*Step 2: The anatomical localization* is the muscle.

*Step 3: Pathological diagnosis* is inflammatory myopathy, i.e. "polymyositis".

*Step 4: Etiological diagnosis*—Polymyositis was of a short duration, only for a few days immediately following a febrile illness. it is more likely to be viral polymyositis than immune-mediated.

The investigation of choice to confirm the anatomical localization is CK and EMG. CK was 2650 I.U and EMG was normal.

***Diagnosis:*** Viral polymyositis.

Viral polymyositis is a self-limiting illness. In spite of high CK levels the EMG characteristically is normal or is marginally abnormal unlike in immune-mediated polymyositis. With a short course of steroids, there was remarkable recovery.

***Case History:*** A 52-year-old female presented with history of painful proximal muscle weakness of *upper limbs* bilaterally in the form of difficulty to comb, wear the blouse, and pick up articles from the top shelf, of four weeks duration. In the 2nd week of illness she also experienced difficulty in taking the food to the mouth but no difficulty to mix food, buttoning, etc. In the 3rd week of illness she had difficulty to get up from Indian toilet seat which worsened over the next seven days. However once she stood up, she could walk fairly normally. She developed skin rash over the forearms and the face in the 3rd week; simultaneously she had difficulty to lift her head off the bed and difficulty to swallow but no nasal regurgitation.

Examination showed proximal muscle weakness, 2/5 power, in all the four limbs with preserved tendon reflexes and normal sensory examination.

### Clinical Diagnosis

*Step 1*: *Neurological deficit*—Proximal muscle weakness of upper and lower limbs, neck flexors, and dysphagia with preserved sensory and tendon reflexes.

*Step 2*: *Anatomical localization*—Muscles – myopathy.

*Step 3*: *Pathological diagnosis*—Subacute, progressive over a period of four weeks—inflammatory—Immune-mediated polymyositis.

*Step 4*: *Etiological diagnosis*—In view of the skin rash over the forearm and infraorbital region immune - mediated dermatomyositis.

Further history revealed that one year earlier she was diagnosed to have carcinoma ovary for which she was operated and radiotherapy given.

**Final diagnosis:** Polymyositis in relation to carcinoma ovary.

The prognosis depends on the types of polymyositis (Table 17.8).

### Table 17.8: Types of polymyositis.

- Polymyositis
- Dermatomyositis
- Polymyositis as part of systemic collagen disease, e.g. rheumatoid arthritis, SLE (systemic lupus erythematosus)
- Polymyositis in association with carcinoma, particularly ovary, lung etc.

Specific cause of Polymyositis helps for proper management and prognosis.

*Case History*: A 50-year-old obese female consulted for difficulty in walking and inability to get up from squatting position for the previous 3 years. She was seen initially by an orthopedic surgeon who got the imaging of the knee joints done and quickly advised bilateral total knee replacement with a diagnosis of osteoarthritis of knee. Clinical examination showed no evidence of pain in the knee joint even with full flexion! The difficulty in getting up from squatting was not due to pain in the knee joints but due to proximal muscle weakness. The waddling gait which is common in both osteoarthritis knee and myopathy can be distinguished by the pain in the knee joint with active/passive movement.

Further investigations confirmed limb girdle muscular dystrophy.

**Final diagnosis:** Limb girdle muscular dystrophy.

**Message:** Diagnosis should be based on clinical examination and not by looking at the image of knee joints.

Inclusion body myositis may be confused with polymyositis (Table 17.9).

#### Table 17.9: Inclusion body myositis—clinical features.

- Age of onset—55–60 years
- Sex—F>M
- Inflammatory myopathy
- Chronic progressive muscle weakness, asymmetrical
- Distal and proximal muscles
- Quadriceps, dorsiflexors of ankle (foot drop), finger flexors, commonly affected
- Marked atrophy of forearm muscles
- CK normal to mild elevation
- Treatment—Generally resistant to all therapies
  Corticosteroids, immunosuppressive therapy, IV IgG to be tried.

Chasing the blood cholesterol levels in healthy individuals and prescribing statins is fairly prevalent. Statin induced myopathy should be recognized to change the drug and give relief to patient (Table 17.10).

#### Table 17.10: Statin induced myopathy.

- Myalgia, fatigue, cramps
- Muscle weakness (myositis)
- Occasionally rhabdomyolysis
- Diagnosis—elevated CK, more than 10 times
- Treatment—stop statin, recovery may take 2–3 months

**Management**
Use another statin or non-statin lipid lowering agent
- Pravastatin, fluvastatin less likely to cause myopathy
- Simvastatin more often causes myopathy

Polymyalgia rheumatica is seen in elderly and is an eminently treatable disorder (Table 17.11).

#### Table 17.11: Polymyalgia rheumatica—clinical features.

- Age above 50 years
- Pain and stiffness of shoulder, low back, and lower limbs
- ESR increased usually above 50 mm at the end of one hour
- Associated giant cell arteritis likely
- Treatment—excellent response to steroids, also works as therapeutic test

# 18

# Pins/Needles in Feet

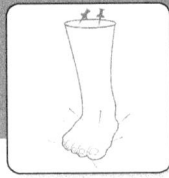

Tingling, numbness, paresthesia, "jum jum" sensation are some of the common complaints in the OPD for which a quick prescription is doled out with a combination of B complex. A good history taking – the basics of clinical medicine – is imperative (Table 18.1).

### Table 18.1: What is not peripheral neuropathy?
- *Intermittent* numbness, 'jum jum' sensation
- Numbness in one half of the body
- Numbness of one limb

Peripheral nerves have three components—sensory, motor, and autonomic and manifestations are positive and negative symptoms.

## Sensory Symptoms

*Positive sensory symptoms* consist of pain, dysesthesia, paresthesia, tingling, burning, pricking. Once the sensory fibers are destroyed it leads to *negative symptoms* like numbness, loss of appreciation of touch, hot and cold, touch of the clothes the person is wearing, inability to appreciate the firmness of the ground. In advanced stages, it may lead to trophic ulcers. In patients who have disabling sensory symptoms like burning pain disturbing the sleep, are now happy that the pain has disappeared, *it may be good or bad,* good if the sensory signs are normal—which means restoration of nerve functions, bad if the patient has lost the ability to appreciate pain, touch and temperature all of which point to advancement of neuropathy.

*Positive posterior column sensory symptoms* consist of band-like constriction around the toe or the foot, the *negative symptom* is imbalance sensory ataxia—which worsen in the dark.

## Motor Symptoms

The *positive motor symptoms* consist of twitching, fasciculations, myokymia. However all these are unusual in the common varieties of peripheral neuropathy. The *negative motor symptoms* consist of motor weakness, wasting in distal muscles with inability to perform finer movements of the hands, difficulty to grip slippers. If one is *aware* of slippers slipping off the feet it is motor weakness; if *unaware* it is sensory deficit.

## Autonomic Symptoms

Impotence, bladder, bowel dysfunction, orthostatic hypotension (Table 18.2)
The clinical features also depend on the type of fiber involvement.

Table 18.2: Peripheral neuropathy—clinical features.

| Clinical feature | Irritative stage | Paralytic stage |
| --- | --- | --- |
| Sensory | Tingling<br>Burning pain<br>Dysesthesia<br>Hyperesthesia<br>Hyperalgesia | Numbness<br>Loss of sensation—pain, touch, temperature |
| Posterior column | Band-like sensation across toe, leg | Sensory ataxia |
| Motor | Cramps, fasciculations | Weakness, atrophy |
| Autonomic dysfunction | Heat intolerance, sweating | Impotence, bladder, bowel dysfunction; Orthostatic hypotension |
| Ankle reflex | — | Absent |

### Small Fiber Neuropathy

(Involvement of unmyelinated or small myelinated fibers)
- Pain, touch, temperature impaired
- Preserved tendon reflexes

### Large Fiber Neuropathy

(Involvement of large myelinated fibers)
- Joint position, vibration sense impaired
- Sensory ataxia
- Absent tendon reflexes

### Diagnostic Approach to Peripheral Neuropathy

### Is this Peripheral Neuropathy?

A clinical diagnosis of peripheral neuropathy is valid if any or all of the symptoms mentioned above are present.

This is further strengthened by physical signs of glove and stocking sensory disturbances (pin, cotton touch, sense of vibration) and weakness and wasting of distal muscles, if motor component is affected. The ankle jerk is usually absent.

Further diagnostic workup depends on the following observations. (Table 18.3).

**Table 18.3: Pattern of involvement in neuropathy.**

- Mononeuropathy/plexopathy/mononeuropathy multiplex
- Unilateral/bilateral; symmetrical/asymmetrical, proximal/distal
- Pure motor, pure sensory/mixed
- Upper limb predominance/lower limb predominance
- Associated autonomic or cranial nerve involvement
- Onset—acute/subacute/chronic; relapsing – remitting

The pattern has to be diligently looked for as it is a *gateway to the possible final diagnosis*.

The etiological causes are specific to the pattern of neuropathy.

The common type of neuropathy is bilateral symmetrical distal sensory/sensory motor neuropathy (Table 18.4).

**Table 18.4: Clinical features of symmetric distal neuropathy.**

- Symptoms—Tingling, numbness, burning paresthesia, hyperesthesia, motor weakness of hands and feet; bilateral symmetric distal
- Signs—Diminished sensations—pin, touch, temperature
- Diminished/absent ankle reflex
- Causes—Symmetric distal neuropathies are due to *several systemic disorders*. The commonest being diabetes (Table 18.5)

**Table 18.5: Common systemic causes for peripheral neuropathy.**

- Deficiency disorders—Vitamin B1, B6, B12
- Endocrine—Hypothyroidism
- Metabolic—Diabetes
- Toxic—Alcohol, heavy metals
- Drugs—INH, vincristine, digoxin, lithium
- Autoimmune disorders

The common variety of peripheral neuropathy is diabetic in origin, simply because diabetes is the common medical disorder affecting a large population. Diabetic neuropathy typically is bilateral, symmetrical and distal, affecting first the feet as the longest axons are in the lower limbs and then as the symptoms progress to mid calf region, distal part of upper limbs are affected.

**Case History:** A 56-year-old female long standing diabetic, complained of burning paresthesia in the feet disturbing her sleep. Examination showed hyperesthesia over both feet and absent ankle jerks. There was no motor weakness.

**Diagnosis:** Diabetic sensory neuropathy.

*Nerve conduction studies are superfluous and academic in nature.*

**Case History:** A 65-year-old female long standing diabetic complained of difficulty in walking due to imbalance, which became worse in the dark.

On probing she told that her slippers slip off without her knowledge. She did not have tingling, numbness or paresthesia at any time. On examination there were no motor or sensory signs, ankle reflex was absent bilaterally and here the focused neurological examination consists of elicitation of Romberg's sign, i.e. patient is asked to stand with feet together, when her eyes were open she was stable, but with eyes closed, she became unstable to the extent of falling, confirming sensory ataxia. In addition absence of vibration and joint position point to posterior column dysfunction.

*Diagnosis*: Sensory ataxia due to diabetic sensory neuropathy (posterior column sensory dysfunction).

**Message:** Peripheral neuropathy can *manifest only* as sensory ataxia without paresthesia, loss of sensory functions to cotton touch, pin.

Certain clinical features distinguish neuropathy of systemic causes from local causes (Table 18.6).

### Table 18.6: When is neuropathy not due to systemic cause?
- Unilateral, e.g. brachial plexopathy
- Bilateral but asymmetric
- Starting or predominantly in upper limbs
- Confined to one nerve (mononeuropathy)
- Proximal more than distal

*In essence only distal symmetric distribution starting in lower limbs is of systemic origin.*

Any other pattern deviating from this is due to other causes, e.g. vasculitis, infective, compressive, infiltrative. Diabetes causes symmetric neuropathy due to metabolic disorder, as well as myeloencephalopathy due to muscle complication.

### Mononeuropathy
Here a single nerve trunk is affected. If acute it is due to a vascular cause and if subacute/chronic it is due to a compressive cause.

Diabetic vasculitic neuropathy causes mononeuropathy affecting ulnar, median, radial, lateral popliteal nerves.

### Carpal Tunnel Syndrome
**Case History**: A 60-year-old female non-diabetic complained of disturbed sleep in the night, waking up in the early hours with uncomfortable dysesthesias in her right hand which initially she attributed to sleeping with her head on the right hand. As the symptoms persisted she sought a consultation. First thing that strikes is that the patient has a positive sensory symptom that is localized to thumb and index finger. The anatomical localization is median nerve. Some patients have wasting of abductor pollicis brevis confirming the involvement of motor component of median nerve.

***Diagnosis:*** Right carpal tunnel syndrome—chronic compression of median nerve.

***Investigation:*** Median nerve conduction block, at carpal tunnel.

Foot drop can be due to an UMN lesion, LMN lesion at the level of root (L5-S1) due to disc prolapse or LMN lesion due to lateral popliteal nerve paralysis at the neck of fibula. Ankle jerk forms a crucial physical sign to differentiate the three. Foot drop with absent ankle jerk is a root lesion (L5-S1) as the reflex pathway travels through these roots. Foot drop with intact ankle jerk is seen in lateral popliteal nerve palsy as it supplies only the dorsi flexors of the ankle but does not participate in the reflex pathway. Foot drop with exaggerated ankle jerk is UMN lesion (Table 18.7).

**Table 18.7: Differential diagnosis of foot drop.**

|  | Lateral popliteal nerve palsy | L5 radiculopathy | UMN—Spinal cord |
|---|---|---|---|
| Distribution of weakness | Dorsiflexors of ankle | Dorsiflexors of ankle | Distal, entire limb |
| Tone | Hypo | Hypo | Hyper |
| Ankle jerk | Normal | Absent/hypo | Exaggerated |
| Plantar reflex | Flexor | Flexor | Extensor |
| Sensory findings | Normal/varying sensory loss dorsum of foot | May be impaired | Normal/impaired in other limb |
| Associated features | Nil | Backache along L5 distribution | Spasticity of ipsilateral limb |

## How to differentiate sensory symptoms of peripheral nerve localization from spinal cord localization?

As long as the symptoms are confined to the lower limbs, distally, consisting of numbness and tingling, it could mean involvement of peripheral nerve, root, or even spinal cord (sensory tracts). What definitely points to a peripheral origin is shock like sensation, burning pain aggravated by touching of the clothes so much so that they cannot wear socks or even cover themselves with a bed sheet. All these point to the involvement of peripheral sensory involvement. Characteristically the sensory symptoms ascend up to the mid-calf and then jump to the fingers and hand (length dependent neuropathy), evading thighs. This pattern is diagnostic of peripheral neuropathy. A situation where tingling continues to spread upward from the feet involving the entire lower limbs and the lower abdomen suggests spinal cord localization (Table 18.8).

**Table 18.8: Differentiation of sensory symptoms of peripheral neuropathy and myelopathy.**

| Symptoms | Peripheral neuropathy | Myelopathy |
|---|---|---|
| ❏ Tingling numbness | + | + |
| ❏ Hyperalgesia | + | – |
| ❏ Hyperesthesia | + | – |
| ❏ Sensory symptoms | Distal | Entire lower limbs |
| ❏ Ankle jerk | Absent | Brisk |
| ❏ Plantar reflex | Flexor | Extensor |

**Investigations in peripheral neuropathy:** The investigation of choice for the anatomical localization is nerve conduction studies (NCV).

Nerve conduction may be normal in frank neuropathies and abnormal in asymptomatic patients and also depends a lot on the experience of the operator (Table 18.9).

**Table 18.9: Utility of nerve conduction studies.**

- ❏ Confirming the diagnosis of neuropathy. In the process excluding the disorders of myoneural junction and muscle
- ❏ The type of neuropathy—sensory/motor or mixed
- ❏ The pathological type—demyelinating or axonal or conduction block
- ❏ Symmetric/asymmetric
- ❏ Mono/polyneuropathy

*Pitfalls of Depending on Nerve Conduction Study*

The patient may have typical burning dysesthesias in the feet, and one expects to find an absent ankle jerk, but surprisingly it may be in intact. Even the nerve conduction studies show normal results. One should not discard the diagnosis but bank on the symptoms. This is because the sensory symptoms are due to unmyelinated or small myelinated fibers which do not take part in the nerve conduction or in the ankle reflex pathways. However if the symptoms are due to posterior column dysfunction like sensory ataxia one would definitely expect absent ankle jerks and delayed conduction velocities. In diabetics and elderly patients the ankle reflex may be absent, even though there are no symptoms or signs of peripheral neuropathy. Nerve conduction studies may be normal in small fiber neuropathy and abnormal *in asymptomatic individuals* (diabetic, elderly).

Similarly, median nerve conduction block at the wrist (carpal tunnel syndrome) is often observed in asymptomatic individuals, hence the investigative reports are *relevant only if correlating with clinical diagnosis*.

## INVESTIGATIONS FOR ETIOLOGICAL DIAGNOSIS

Basic—Hemogram, blood sugar, B12, folic acid, renal, hepatic profile.

Add on—Protein electrophoresis HIV, ANA, dsDNA, ACE,
Vasculitic profile: nerve biopsy in select cases (Table 18.10).

| Table 18.10: Indications for nerve biopsy. |
|---|
| ❏ Hansen's disease |
| ❏ Vasculitic neuropathy |
| ❏ Amyloid neuropathy |
| ❏ Hereditary neuropathy |

### Psychogenic Causes

Intermittent fluctuating numbness of one half of the body particularly in women is a common psychogenic complaint. Sensory symptoms which are *transient, changing locations,* inconsistent and of *long duration* not *affecting daily* activities point to psychogenic origin. Elderly patients often complain of sensory symptoms in one limb or one half of body and reassurance that these symptoms are non specific and *will not lead to stroke* is more satisfying than a flurry of investigations, because they are worried that the sensory symptoms are the forerunner of stroke! I reassure them saying that "stroke strikes suddenly: and it does not send messages!" So note that any "jum jum" sensation is not neuropathy.

***Case History:*** A 30-year-old female complains of intermittent numbness of left lower limb of three months duration. MR lumbar spine showed L4, 5 disc prolapse and she was referred for opinion on possibility of surgical management.

Further history revealed that the numbness fluctuated more in the later part of the day and on probing further she mentioned that she also had other fluctuating symptoms like numbness of left upper limb and chronic headache.

Step 1: *Neurological deficit*—Total loss of sensation in the left upper and lower limb with normal motor power and gait.

Step 2: *Anatomical localization*—Total loss of sensation, means sensory nerve root affecting the entire lower and upper limb which is not possible with history of fluctuating symptoms.

***Diagnosis*** is psychogenic—functional- which required no further investigation. Patient was referred to a psychiatrist.

### Symptomatic Management of Sensory Neuropathy

The drugs used for positive sensory symptoms like burning paresthesia, disturbing pain, tingling are tricyclic antidepressants (amitriptyline) and antiepileptic drugs (carbamazepine, gabapentin).

These are NOT useful in negative sensory symptoms like numbness, loss of sensation.

## HANSEN'S DISEASE

Hansen's disease being less common, is usually not thought of. However, it is an eminently treatable condition, so one should not miss it.

Hansen's disease is classified into tuberculoid, borderline, lepromatous. Neuropathy is commonly seen in tuberculoid. Lepromatous type is reflection of low immunity and bacilli can be detected in skin biopsy.

The diagnosis of Hansen's neuropathy can be confirmed by appropriate nerve biopsy which shows inflammatory changes with lepra bacilli. The treatment is for 6 months to 2 years.

**Case History:** A 35-year-old male complained of loss of sensation over the dorsal aspect of right hand and middle finger. Nerve conduction done showed evidence of "carpal tunnel syndrome".

Clinical examination showed depigmented hypoesthetic large patch over the dorsum of the hand extending to the middle finger.

**Diagnosis:** "Hansen's disease". Nerve conduction showing carpal tunnel syndrome is *incidental* because the median nerve which traverses through the carpal tunnel does not supply the skin of dorsum of the hand!

**Message:** Investigation without a clinical diagnosis may take you up the wrong path!

**Case History:** A 56-year-old male presented with history of numbness of right face of one year duration and numbness of the right foot since six months and inability to close right eye since three months. He was on antidepressants for a long period of time. He had already undergone extensive investigations including MR brain, cervical spine and LS spine all of which were normal. On examination he had partial LMN facial palsy with reduced pin sensation and greatly thickened great auricular nerve, ulnar nerve and right lateral popliteal nerve.

**Message:** Partial facial palsy means one of the branches of facial nerve is affected and NOT the nerve trunk as in Bell's palsy. Hansen's disease does not involve the nerve trunk. Patchy sensory loss over face is suggestive of sensory nerve twigs involvement, NOT trigeminal nerve trunk.

**Diagnosis:** Hansen's disease.

Thickened nerves are commonly seen in ulnar, lateral popliteal nerves. The thickened cutaneous nerves are observed in great auricular nerve, dorsal cutaneous branch of ulnar nerve and cutaneous branch of radial nerve.

Hansen's neuropathy is predominantly sensory or sensory motor and manifests as mononeuropathy/mononeuropathy multiplex.

### Lateral Popliteal Nerve Palsy

**Case History:** A 35-year-old male diabetic of 10 years duration had abrupt onset of difficulty in walking with left foot. On examination there was left foot drop with *intact ankle jerk* with no sensory impairment.

*Step 1:* Neurological deficit—Left ankle dorsiflexor paresis.
*Step 2:* Anatomical localization—Lateral popliteal nerve.
*Step 3:* Pathological diagnosis—Abrupt onset—vascular—lateral popliteal nerve infarct.
*Step 4:* Etiological diagnosis—Diabetic vasculitis.

**Diagnosis:** Lateral popliteal nerve palsy.

# CHAPTER 19

# Tremors

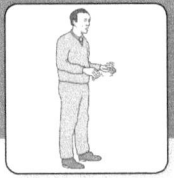

Tremors consist of rhythmic involuntary movements of limbs, head, jaw, and voice.

Tremors are a common complaint seen in the OPD and if it is a senior citizen he is always worried about whether it is Parkinson's disease!

The different types of tremors are listed in Table 19.1

### Table 19.1: Types of tremor.
a. Resting tremors, e.g. Parkinson's disease
b. Action tremor—postural tremor, kinetic tremor
c. Intention tremor/goal directed tremor, e.g. cerebellar dysfunction
d. Task specific tremor—writing tremor
e. Isometric tremors (orthostatic tremor)

a. ***Resting tremor:*** Tremors are seen in the hands when it is resting. It starts unilaterally and subsequently spreads to the other side. The tremors get arrested when an activity starts, like holding a glass of water and restart when the limb is resting. Typically it is seen in *Parkinson's disease*. There may be additional features like unilateral rigidity, bradykinesia and low volume speech.

## Management

Mere presence of tremors *does not require treatment* if it is not disturbing the daily activities, e.g. an elderly retired school teacher with tremors in the left hand, who can continue all his activities with the left hand without any difficulty, does not require treatment. However a middle-aged executive who has tremors in the right hand that interferes with writing and signature requires treatment. An anticholinergic like trihexyphenidyl is the drug of choice to suppress tremors and levodopa may be added when required (for further information *see* Chapter 19).

b. **Action tremor:** Occurs during an action involving *voluntary contraction* of muscles (Table 19.2).
   i. Postural (when a person is asked to stretch both his arms in front of his body and hold it).
   ii. Kinetic tremors during the movement of the limb, e.g. while drinking water from a glass, tremors occur and the water spills.

### Table 19.2: The common causes of action tremors.

- Anxiety
- Chronic alcohol intake
- Thyrotoxicosis
- Hypoglycemia
- Hepatic encephalopathy

All the above are treatable, once the underlying cause is attended to. The following drugs may induce tremors (Table 19.3):

### Table 19.3: Drug-induced tremors.

- Valproic acid
- Lithium
- Salbutamol
- Cyclosporine
- Amphetamine
- Theophylline
- Nicotine
- Cinnarizine

***Benign essential tremor*** is a type of action tremor with no known cause—also known as essential tremor (like essential hypertension). Benign is a misnomer as it does affect the lifestyle and daily activities, but it is benign in the sense that it "wont kill"! The tremors are bilateral, symmetric, postural or kinetic and can also involve the *head (titubation), jaw and voice*. Characteristically the tremors subside with alcohol intake but do not try to suggest this to patients as in one of my patients, over a period of time, the essential tremors subsided giving rise to alcohol induced tremors!

In about 50% it is inherited as an autosomal dominant trait, in which case it starts at a young age; otherwise it usually starts after 40 years of age. It is called familial tremor when there is family history.

Mild tremors of the hand do not cause any problems except for the signature but as the tremors increase the person may have difficulty in holding a plate or a glass of water. Head tremors are more of a social embarrassment than any physical disability.

**Treatment of essential tremors** is suggested only when the tremors are causing some disability. If the patient says he does not have any difficulty to perform the daily activities, there is no need to start treatment. At times the patient says that when he meets a new person or when guests arrive the tremors become obvious and embarrassing. In such cases *situational treatment* by administering propranolol 20-40 mg two hours before the event, will take care of these situational tremors. When the tremors are persistently affecting the daily activities, e.g. in an executive who has to sign several cheques and conduct several meetings it definitely needs continuous treatment.

The pharmacological treatment consists of beta blockers, in particular, propranolol starting with a small dose of 20 mg in the morning and increased steadily to adequate dosage of 40-120 mg per day. When propranolol is ineffective or contraindicated, primidone (mysoline) is the next drug of choice. As it causes drowsiness the drug should be started at a very low dose—¼ of a 250 mg tablet). If ¼ tablet is not tolerated, start with 1/6 of a tablet and increase progressively every week to the required dose. The other drugs used are clonazepam, topiramate and gabapentin. When the pharmacological treatment fails botulinum toxin injection (Botox) and occasionally in severe cases surgery, i.e. deep brain stimulation of the thalamus, is advocated.

Essential tremors should be differentiated from Parkinson's tremors (Table 19.4).

Table 19.4: Differential features of essential tremors and Parkinson's tremors.

|  | Essential tremors | Parkinson's tremors |
|---|---|---|
| ❏ Resting | Absent | Present |
| ❏ Postural/action (arms extended) | Present | Absent |
| ❏ Attempting to do work | Increases | Disappears |
| ❏ Age at onset | Bimodal 15–20 yr and 50–70 year | 55–75 year |
| ❏ Distribution | Bilateral symmetric | Unilateral |
| ❏ Associated signs | Head tremors<br>Voice tremors<br>Jaw tremors | Rigidity<br>Bradykinesia<br>Dysarthria |
| ❏ Treatment | Propranolol/primidone | Anticholinergics |

c. *Intention tremor (goal directed tremor):* Here the tremors are obvious when the target is being reached, like picking up a glass from the table and as it reaches the mouth the tremors become obvious and coarse. This is seen in cerebellar dysfunction.

d. *Task specific:* These tremors appear only for a particular task, the commonest being the writing tremor (for further information *see* Chapter 12).

e. *Isometric (orthostatic)* tremors occur when the muscles contract without movement, e.g. where a person feels discomfort in the legs, while standing, due to tremors in the calf muscles *which can be felt.*

*Case History:* A 35-year-old female complained of pain and extreme discomfort in both calf muscles on standing which was relieved on walking or sitting. The diagnosis is entirely on clinical history and the tremors of calf muscles can be felt when the person is standing.

*Diagnosis:* "Orthostatic tremors" and the treatment is clonazepam.

# 20. Parkinson's Disease

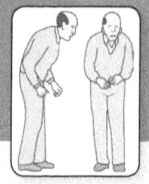

*I am having tremors, Doctor do I have Parkinson's disease?*
Many patients with tremors consult with the above question.

The tremors in Parkinson's disease occur at rest (resting tremors) and disappears on movement. Essential tremors on the other hand appears during movement and disappear at rest (for differential diagnosis of tremors *see* Chapter 19).

*What is Parkinsonism and Parkinson's disease? (Tables 20.1 and 20.2)*

### Table 20.1: Parkinsonism is a syndrome consisting of:
- Rigidity
- Bradykinesia
- Tremor
- Gait disorder

Parkinson's disease is a *definitive diagnosis* of the above features.

### Table 20.2: Parkinsonism—differential diagnosis.
- I Idiopathic Parkinson's disease
- II Vascular Parkinsonism
- III Secondary Parkinsonism (secondary to drugs)
- IV Parkinson's plus/atypical Parkinsonism

## I. IDIOPATHIC PARKINSON'S DISEASE

It is the second most common neurodegenerative disorder (after Alzheimer's) which is due to progressive degeneration of dopaminergic nigral cells and intracellular inclusions of Lewy bodies. Symptoms occur when 70-80% of neurons become dysfunctional (Table 20.3).

### Table 20.3: Diagnostic features of Parkinson's disease.
- Unilateral onset
- Tremors at rest
- Bradykinesia
- Rigidity
- Gait disorder
- Excellent response to levodopa
- Slow progression

## Parkinson's Disease

### How to confirm the diagnosis?
Parkinson's disease is a clinical diagnosis.
Investigations—Nil; no laboratory tests, no imaging
Clinical neurology is still supreme!

In clinical practice any tremors are mistaken as Parkinson's disease (overdiagnosis) and Parkinson's disease presenting with bradykinesia and rigidity but *no tremors* are mistaken for UMN hemiparesis (underdiagnosis).

***Case History*:** A 45-year-old male presented with difficulty in writing, buttoning, mixing food and also had pain in the right upper limb—both proximal and distal. Examination showed stiffness of right upper and lower limb with no tremors. The clinician diagnosed it as right-sided hemiparesis with pain in the neck and shoulder and advised an MR cervical spine which revealed C5-6 disc prolapse, and was operated upon. Over the next few weeks the symptoms worsened and when reviewed, his symptoms were due to rigidity of Parkinson's disease and not due to spasticity!

***Diagnosis*:** Parkinson's disease.

**Message:** A basic clinical approach to differentiate spasticity and rigidity was required and radiological findings, were incidental and not causative!

***Case History*:** A 68-year-old male, an accountant by occupation had difficulty in writing, mixing food, shaving, over the past six months and as the symptoms were progressive he stopped writing. He was asked to do tests like MR brain, MR cervical spine, carotid Doppler and ENMG!

What did the clinical examination show? Stiffness of wrist and fingers—extrapyramidal rigidity and when asked to write he showed typical micrographia—the words becoming smaller and smaller and illegible.

**Diagnosis:** Right hemi-Parkinson's disease (rigidity only, no tremors).

***Message*:** Remember to examine what the patient is complaining of—here it is difficulty to write—so ask him to write and observe.

**Parkinson's disease—Management:** The cause being—dopamine deficiency, management is by replacement therapy with levodopa, but levodopa administration over a period of 5-10 years becomes less effective and also results in unacceptable side effects (Table 20.4).

### Table 20.4: Pharmacotherapy in Parkinson's disease.
- MAO—Inhibitors—Selegiline, rasagiline
- Dopaminergic drugs—Pramipexole, ropinirole
- Anticholinergics—Trihexyphenidyl
- Levodopa metabolized via two pathways:
  - Decarboxylation—blocked by carbidopa, benserazide
  - COMT (Catechol-O-methyltransferase)—COMT inhibitors—Entacapone, Tolcapone
- Amantadine
- Vitamin E, coenzyme not useful

***Management Goals*:** Symptom relief with minimal adverse effects.

### Parkinson's disease — When to start treatment?

*Diagnosis Does Not Mean Start Treatment*

a. If there is no functional impairment, reassure the patient that there is a treatment available but it will be administered only if the symptoms are interfering with daily activities. One can start selegiline 10 mg or Rasagiline 1 mg which may reduce the progress of the disease in addition to mild symptomatic relief.
b. If the activities of daily living are affected by tremors then anticholinergic—trihexyphenidyl (pacitane 2 mg ½ tds to be increased over a week or two to 1 tds).
c. If the activities of daily living are affected by bradykinesia or rigidity then —dopa agonist—ropinirole, pramipexole to be started.
d. If there is sufficient functional impairment in spite of dopaminergic drugs then only levodopa-carbidopa combination should be started. Start with a lower dose and gradually titrate upwards to the required dosage.

Idiopathic Parkinson's disease has much better prognosis and responds very well to levodopa for the first 5 years and moderately for the next 5 years, while Parkinson's syndrome either does not respond or responds poorly to therapy.

*Surgery in Parkinson's Disease*

Earlier ablative surgery was resorted to which is not done anymore. Currently deep brain stimulation (DBS) of subthalamic nucleus, globus pallidus interna and thalamus is performed (Tables 20.5 and 20.6).

**Table 20.5: Indications for DBS.**
- *Good response* to levodopa
- Disabling on/off periods
- Disabling dyskinesia, tremors

**Table 20.6: Contraindications for DBS.**
- No response to levodopa
- Cognitive, psychiatric disability
- Postural instability

Initially Parkinson's disease was thought to be purely a movement disorder affecting the motor system, however in recent times several non-motor symptoms are being recognized, many of them seen in the later stages (Table 20.7).

## Table 20.7: Non-motor symptoms in Parkinson's disease.

- Neuropsychiatric features:
  Anxiety, panic attacks, depression, hallucinations, illusions, delusions
- Cognitive deterioration—dementia.
- Autonomic dysfunction:
  Orthostatic hypotension, constipation, urinary dysfunction (urgency, retention), sexual dysfunction, excessive sweating, seborrhea, sialorrhea.
- Sleep disorders—Insomnia, REM behavior disorder, restless legs syndrome, periodic limb movements in sleep, excessive daytime sleepiness
- Sensory dysfunction—hyposmia (i.e. loss of sense of smell), pain, fatigue.

## II. VASCULAR PARKINSONISM

Vascular Parkinsonism has different manifestation and prognosis (Table 20.8).

## Table 20.8: Clinical features of vascular Parkinsonism.

- Due to cerebrovascular ischemia, also referred as lower body Parkinsonism.
- Multi-infarct state, diffuse white matter lesion
- No tremors, no bradykinesia
- Difficulty to walk—postural instability
- Wide-based gait
- Pyramidal signs
- Poor response to levodopa

**Case History:** A 60-year-old female was brought with a history of difficulty in walking and difficulty in finer movements of right hand like brushing and writing of one month duration. She was referred with a diagnosis of right hemi-Parkinson's disease. However history revealed acute onset with some improvement.

Diagnostic steps:

*Step 1: Neurological deficit*—Rigidity of right upper and lower limbs with mild tremors - extrapyramidal disorder.

*Step 2: Anatomical localization*—Left basal ganglia.

*Step 3: Pathological diagnosis*—In view of acute onset, vascular cause.

*Step 4: Etiological diagnosis*—Lacunar infarcts in basal ganglia due to hypertension.

**Diagnosis:** Acute hemi-Parkinsonism.

**Message:** It is the history which differentiated idiopathic Parkinson's disease from abrupt onset acute vascular parkinsonism which has good prognosis with spontaneous recovery. This is different from chronic vascular parkinsonism described above (Table 20.9).

**Table 20.9: Differentiation of idiopathic Parkinson's disease, vascular Parkinsonism, normal pressure hydrocephalus.**

|  | Parkinson's disease | Vascular Parkinsonism | Normal pressure hydrocephalus |
| --- | --- | --- | --- |
| Gait | Narrow base | Wide base | Wide base |
| Upper limbs | Affected | Normal | Normal |
| Speech | Affected | Normal | Normal |
| Lower limbs | Affected | Affected | Affected |
| Tremors | + | - | - |
| Course of illness | Progressive | Minor fluctuations | Progressive |
| UMN signs | - | + | +/- |

For more information on normal pressure hydrocephalus refer Chapter 20.

## III. SECONDARY PARKINSONISM

Parkinson's features are secondary to various causes (Table 20.10).

**Table 20.10: Causes of secondary Parkinsonism.**

- Drug-induced—antipsychotics, risperidone, haloperidol (Table 20.11)
  - Antiemetics—Phenothiazine, metoclopramide
  - Antivertigo—Cinnarizine
- Manganese, carbon monoxide toxicity
- Encephalitis, head injury
- Hypoxia, hypothermia
- Wilson's disease
- Normal pressure hydrocephalus

**Table 20.11: Clinical features of drug-induced Parkinsonism.**

- Rigidity
- Symmetric onset
- Static course
- Associated akathisia, dyskinesia

Occasionally when there is a confusion to differentiate idiopathic Parkinson's disease from drug-induced, one can use DaT-SPECT (dopamine transport) imaging. In drug-induced Parkinsonism it will be normal while in idiopathic Parkinson's disease it will be abnormal (low uptake).

**Case History:** A 52-year-old female hypertensive, diabetic was admitted for repeated vomiting for previous 24 hours which was stopped with appropriate medicines. However, 48 hours later she became "zombie-like". MR brain and EEG done were normal. Clinical examination showed Parkinson's features with rigidity of all four limbs and slow gait. Prior to the hospitalization she was very active and ambulant. The *acute* Parkinson's features were due to the antiemetic drug prescribed which recovered with IV Phenergan.

***Diagnosis:*** Drug-induced Parkinsonism.

***Message:*** The diagnosis was made by clinical history and not MR brain or EEG!

## IV. ATYPICAL PARKINSONISM (PARKINSON'S PLUS)

Parkinson-plus should be differentiated from Parkinson's disease as the prognosis and management is different, though both are neurodegenerative disorders (Table 20.12).

**Table 20.12: Types of atypical Parkinsonism.**
- Progressive supranuclear palsy (PSP)
- Multisystem atrophy (MSA-C) (MSA-P)
- Corticobasal degeneration (CBD)
- Dementia with Lewy bodies (LBD)

Suspect atypical Parkinsonism if any of the following are seen during first 2–3 years (Table 20.13).

**Table 20.13: Atypical Parkinsonism—clinical features.**
- Symmetric onset
- Poor response to levodopa
- Absence of tremors
- Postural instability
- Frequent falls early in illness
- Dementia
- Hallucinations
- Freezing
- Autonomic dysfunction

***Case History:*** A 52-year-old male presented with progressive difficulty in walking and frequent falls of six months duration. Investigations revealed low serum B12 as the only abnormality. He was administered B12 injection on alternate days and subsequently twice a week over the next two to three months with no improvement. Review showed postural imbalance due to extrapyramidal rigidity of axial muscles—atypical Parkinsonism. *The clue for extrapyramidal rigidity* as a cause of postural imbalance, is that the patient also had *difficulty to turn in the bed, get up from lying to sitting position*, tendency to fall while getting out of chair and quickly turning while walking. In addition vertical eye movements were restricted—probable PSP (progressive supranuclear palsy).

***Management:*** In all patients levodopa preparations should be started. A few of them will respond for a short period. Once the drug is found to have no beneficial effect it should be withdrawn. After that, only supportive therapy is the mainstay of the treatment.

# CHAPTER 21

# Memory Impairment/ Dementia

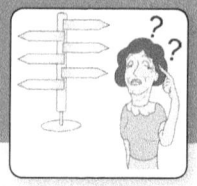

*Doctor I have memory problem. Do you think I have Alzheimer's disease?*
This is a question often asked. With increase in the population of senior citizens there is also an increase in their awareness about dementia.

**Dementia** is diminished mental faculties which include memory, language, personality, social behavior, abstract thinking and visuospatial skills. Brain being the master organ, like a captain of the ship, is the last one to fail and 40% of those who survive beyond 85 years develop dementia. I tell the patient and caregivers "you have heard of liver failure, kidney failure, heart failure—all of which occur at an earlier age;—well, dementia is brain failure. Like the captain of the sinking ship who leaves the ship at the end so also brain failure is the last to occur at the end of our life". The commonest type of dementia is Alzheimer's disease which occurs in 60-70%. One should always recognize treatable dementias, before concluding with a diagnosis of untreatable Alzheimer's disease.

### Observe how the Person with Dementia Presents, when he enters the OPD

Doctor: What is the problem, why have you come?
Patient: I have no problem.
Doctor: Why did you come to the hospital?
Patient: Ask my wife she has brought me. The wife then explains all the clinical features of dementia—forgetfulness, losing his way, not washing after going to the toilet, etc.

This is dementia, patient is blissfully unaware and caregiver bears the brunt.

### Observe how this Person is Presenting

Doctor: What is the problem?
Patient: I am forgetful, my memory is failing. I am afraid i have Alzheimer's disease.
Doctor: Since when?
Patient: About two years.
Doctor: Is it worsening?
Patient: It is the same.

This is not dementia, but is minimal cognitive impairment (MCI) or just anxiety of developing dementia.

## Memory has Four Steps
- Recognition (which requires attention)
- Registration,
- Retention, and
- Recollection.

In dementia the registration is affected because of which activities performed on the same day or preceding days are the first to be forgotten. Remote memory like college days, will be affected much later. When there is difficulty to recognize by name, it is later addition to family—grandchildren's name is forgotten and then gradually the youngest son/daughter, spouse and self. The memory starts getting wiped out from the present time backwards.

Whenever I enquire about memory the immediate response of caregiver is "memory is excellent he can remember his younger days, old friends, etc."

The clinical approach to memory problem is mentioned in Table 21.1.

**Table 21.1: Approach to memory problem.**

**Step 1:** Does the patient have memory problem?
**Step 2:** If yes, is it?
a. Depression/anxiety
b. Minimal cognitive impairment (MCI)
c. Dementia
**Step 3:** If dementia
a. Treatable dementia, e.g.   – B12, folic acid deficiencies
                                  – Hypothyroidism
                                  – Intracranial space occupying lesion
                                  – Autoimmune encephalopathy
                                  – NPH
b. Vascular dementia
c. Degenerative diseases, e.g. Alzheimer's disease
                                  – Frontotemporal dementia
                                  – Lewy body dementia

## STEP 1: DOES THE PATIENT HAVE MEMORY PROBLEM?

A detailed history from the patient and the attendants will sort out the issue. Generally when the patient himself complains, it is unlikely to be dementia. It is either depression or minimal cognitive impairment.

### Are there any Investigations to Confirm the Memory Impairment?

Yes, neuropsychological assessment and lobe function tests done by an experienced clinical neuropsychologist will tell whether the patient has dementia. Also a follow up examination will give an objective evidence of the progression of the disease. However, the catch is that these tests are highly dependent on the patient's attention and cooperation. For example, some patients feel insulted when the psychologist asks "name five cities in India". One patient purposely told the names of neighboring villages because he felt that a man of his caliber was being asked such a stupid question!

In the OPD a brief mini-mental state examination (MMSE) is done which takes about 5-10 minutes and the questionnaire covers registration, attention, calculation, orientation, recall and language and short-term memory. This test requires four frontal lobes two of the examiner's and two of the patient's! (Table 21.2).

**Table 21.2: Mental status examination.**

- Attention—Serial subtraction, reverse digit/month span
- Language—comprehension, naming, repeating
- Visuospatial—To draw face of clock
- Memory—Immediate—Repeat 3 items after 5 minutes
  - — Intermediate
  - — Remote

### STEP 2: PATIENT HAS MEMORY PROBLEM—IS IT DUE TO?

a. **Depression (pseudodementia):** The memory is intact but the person is withdrawn, less communicative, has lack of sleep, loss of appetite. If the patient is cooperative the MMSE will be normal. When in doubt, always prescribe antidepressant drugs and follow-up.

b. **Minimal Cognitive Impairment (MCI):** The forgetfulness is for immediate memory like forgetting where one has kept the car key, purse, letter or forgetting an article which is to be purchased. Above 60 years, 15-20% are affected. Generally, MCI is non-progressive, which means that the same symptoms are experienced for more than 1-2 years, and does not affect day-to-day activities. When prompted the patient is able to identify or recollect the event. However, 10% may progress to dementia as compared to 1% in controls.

c. **Dementia:** The clinical manifestations are like the two sides of a coin (Table 21.3).

**Neurological**—Affecting memory, intelligence, calculation, decision making.

The memory affects daily routine activities like forgetting to take bath, wearing the dress wrongly, asking for food even though the person had just finished eating, unable to recall an important event in the recent past, like a birthday, marriage party, even when prompted. As the disease progresses there is urinary incontinence or passing urine in the wrong place, forgetting the location of the house after going for a walk, and more important even *after reminding, denying the activity.* The symptoms are slowly but relentlessly progressive. The vocabulary is restrictive, repetitive, difficulty in finding words, naming objects and recognizing faces.

**Psychiatric**—Behavioral changes and personality changes. The person who was a recluse, becomes boisterous, with no inhibition, lack of decorum, and has hallucinations.

**Table 21.3: Differentiation between depression, minimal cognitive impairment and dementia.**

|  | Pseudodementia (depression) | Minimal cognitive impairment (MCI) | Dementia |
|---|---|---|---|
| Predominant symptom | Forgetfulness | Forgetfulness | I am OK (no complaints of forgetfulness!) |
| Immediate memory loss | Nil | + | +++ |
| Day to day activities | Unaffected | Unaffected | Affected |
| Progressive memory impairment | – | – | + |
| Associated features | Lack of interest, loss of sleep, loss of appetite, apathy | Quite active but worried about developing dementia | Personality changes, judgment affected, hallucinations |

## STEP 3: DEMENTIA—HOW DO YOU CONFIRM DIAGNOSIS?

Dementia is entirely a clinical diagnosis, with history from the person who is living with the patient supported by neuropsychological evaluation. Nowa-days senior citizens live with a caretaker as their children live abroad. The son may accompany the patient to the OPD when he comes down for a vacation and give second hand and improper information. I always ask "who is taking care of the patient? I want to interview that person for the detailed history". The patient is almost always brought only when he/she is a burden to the family, e.g. the patient may be brought with the complaint that he is passing urine in inappropriate places at home or wetting his bed since one month and is unaware of it. Only when the history is dug out, you literally have to dig deep for it, will you find changes in memory, personality and behavior of more than a year!

On the other hand if dementia develops in a person who is still working and contributing to the family income say a businessman running his own business, the symptoms can be picked up very early. When he starts making mistakes in calculation and money transactions he is immediately brought for consultation! But many of the symptoms in a retired senior citizen who is not working, not earning money, will be passed off as due to "old age".

### 3a: Treatable Dementias

The aim of diagnosing any medical condition is to give relief to the patient by appropriate treatment. The first thing to investigate is whether the patient has treatable dementia which is observed in 15–20%.

The most important clinical point to differentiate non-treatable neurodegenerative disorder from treatable condition is *the speed with which the dementia progresses*. If a proper history is elicited (from the people living and working with him) and it is found that a perfectly normal individual has rapidly progressive dementia, then one should think of a treatable condition and the patient should be thoroughly investigated. In addition, in such patients, language and other faculties are intact; *only the memory is affected* (Table 21.4).

| Table 21.4: Dementia —treatable causes. |
|---|
| ❑ Vitamin B12, B1 folic acid deficiency |
| ❑ Endocrine dysfunction hypothyroid and autoimmune thyroid disorders, adrenal insufficiency, Cushing's syndrome, hypo/hyperparathyroidism |
| ❑ Brain tumors, subdural hematoma, normal pressure hydrocephalus, (MR brain, CSF examination) |
| ❑ Hepatic, renal dysfunction |
| ❑ Drug intoxication, alcohol abuse |
| ❑ Infections—syphilis, HIV, chronic meningitis |

Appropriate investigations to rule out the above treatable causes is mandatory (Fig. 21.1).

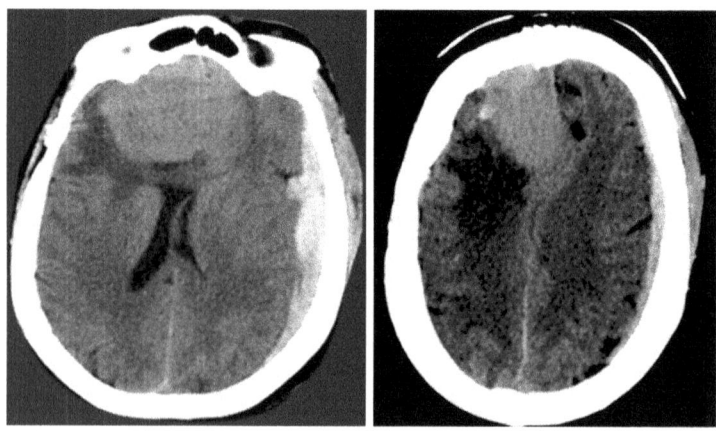

Fig. 21.1: CT brain—meningioma.

*Normal pressure hydrocephalus (NPH)* is a treatable cause of dementia and hence should not be missed (Table 21.5).

| Table 21.5: Normal pressure hydrocephalus (NPH)—clinical features. |
| --- |
| a. Difficulty in walking due to stiffness of lower limb resembling Parkinson's disease |
| b. Cognitive impairment—memory disturbance with slow responses |
| c. Urinary incontinence |

Once the above features are seen in the elderly, MRI of the brain should be done which shows large ventricles (lateral III and to some extent IV ventricle), rounding of the frontal horns. Additionally, CSF flow studies will confirm the presence of NPH (Fig. 21.2).

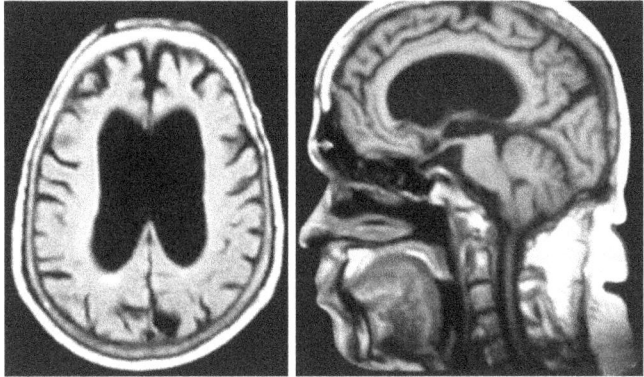

Fig. 21.2: MR brain—normal pressure hydrocephalus.

*Management* consists of drainage LP. 20–30 ml of CSF is drained on alternate days for 3 days and then the change in gait, memory and urinary incontinence is observed. The first to improve is the gait. Over the next few weeks, the CSF reaccumulates and the symptoms recur. The second sitting of drainage LP is useful to reconfirm that the clinical improvement is because of CSF drain. Subsequently as a permanent measure ventriculoperitoneal shunt is advised.

### 3b: Vascular Dementia

Vascular dementia is the second most common type of dementia after Alzheimer's disease. This can be due to: (i) Post-stroke state, (ii) Multi-infarct state. Typically there may be abrupt worsening and *meaningful recovery*. This fluctuating symptomatology in a patient who has vascular disease like hypertension, diabetes, etc. is highly suggestive. In addition, imaging of brain shows chronic ischemic changes. The importance of making a diagnosis of vascular dementia is that with appropriate management of the underlying cause like hypertension, diabetes, dyslipidemia, smoking, etc. the disease can be prevented from worsening unlike in Alzheimer's disease (Table 21.6).

**Table 21.6: Differentiation of vascular dementia from Alzheimer's disease.**

|  | Vascular dementia | Alzheimer's disease |
|---|---|---|
| Symptoms | Present | Absent |
| HBP/diabetes | Present | +/- |
| MR brain | Multiple infarcts | Cerebral atrophy |
| Gait disturbance | Present | Absent |
| Urinary incontinence | Present | Present |
| Pseudobulbar features | Present | Absent |
| Fluctuating symptoms | Present/step wise deterioration | Relentlessly progressive |

### 3c: Dementia—Degenerative Diseases

There are several types of degenerative diseases causing dementia, but the common types are mentioned below (Tables 21.7 and 21.8).

**Table 21.7: Types of neurodegenerative dementia.**

1. Alzheimer's dementia
2. Frontotemporal dementia
3. Lewy body dementia

**Table 21.8: Differentiating features of neurodegenerative dementias.**

|  | AD | FTD | LBD |
|---|---|---|---|
| Memory impairment | +++ | + | + |
| Parkinson's features | – | – | + |
| Visual hallucination | – | + | ++ |
| Auditory hallucination | – | ++ | + |
| Executive dysfunction | – | +++ | – |
| Behavioral changes | – | +++ | – |
| Fluctuating symptoms | – | – | ++ |
| Lesion | Temporoparietal, hippocampal atrophy | Fronto-temporal | Basal ganglia, cerebral cortex |
| Drugs to be avoided | – | Donepezil, rivastigmine | Haloperidol, risperidone, pacitane, dopa agonists |

(AD: Alzheimer's disease; FTD: Frontotemporal dementia; LBD: Lewy body dementia).

In *Alzheimer's dementia* memory impairment is the striking clinical feature. Language, executive functions, behavioral changes add on later. It is the commonest cause of dementia and is relentlessly progressive. MR brain shows cerebral atrophy (Fig. 21.3), but it should be remembered that *mere cerebral atrophy in imaging* is not suggestive of dementia.

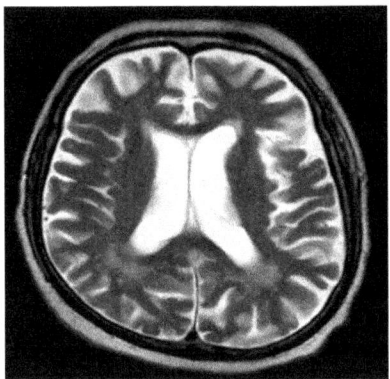 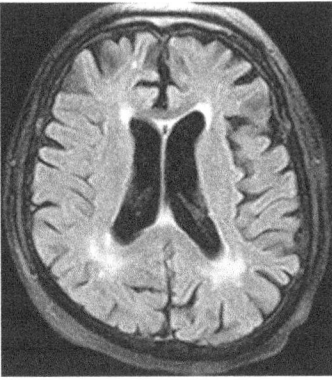

**Fig. 21.3:** MR brain—cerebral atrophy.

Terminally patients are bedridden and blissfully unaware of their problem and the entire burden is on the caregiver.

In frontotemporal dementia, memory is fairly intact but the executive function is affected earlier than memory, with prominent hallucinations and behavioral disturbances.

Lewy body dementia characteristically has fluctuating symptoms and prominent visual hallucinations with associated Parkinson's features, whereas in idiopathic Parkinson's disease dementia occurs much later.

All neurodegenerative dementias progress relentlessly totally dependent for day-to-day activities—feeding, toilet, etc.

### Management of Dementia

After having excluded a treatable cause of dementia very diligently, the management now consists of symptomatic and supportive therapy.

a. For neurological issues like memory there are drugs to improve the acetylcholine level in the brain by using anti-cholinesterase drugs like donepezil, galantamine, rivastigmine. As add on drug NMDA antagonist memantine can be prescribed. If one fails, the other drug may be used and each one should be tried for a period of 3-6 months. During this period if there is a progressive worsening then the medicines can be stopped. Rivastigmine is now available as skin patches for those who cannot swallow it.

b. For psychiatric issues like hallucination, drugs like risperidone, quetiapine are very useful.

c. In Lewy body dementia anticholinesterase drugs, dopaminergic drugs, older antipsychotic drugs, like haloperidol, pacitane group of drugs *should be avoided* as these may exacerbate the symptoms.
d. In frontotemporal dementia, anticholinesterase drugs are not useful.

Apart from the therapeutic intervention, as mentioned above there is a need for an attender to take care of the patient for his day-to-day activities like feeding, bathing, toilet etc. and preventing injuries and accidents like lighting a gas stove and touching a live electric connection. The caregivers must be warned that the patient may open the door at night when everyone is asleep and just disappear. In a way if the patient is not very ambulant due to other reasons like osteoarthritis of knee, mild stroke, etc. it is a blessing in disguise for the caregivers!

For the caregiver it is indeed painful to see that the patient is not appreciating the enormous suffering the caregiver has to undergo in looking after the patient. In other situations like caring for a terminally ill cancer patient, the caregiver is satisfied as the patient acknowledges the attention given but in dementia it is indeed a "thankless job" and this adds to the lack of attention to the patient.

## CAN YOU PREVENT ALZHEIMER'S DISEASE?

Yes, you can reduce the chances by keeping your brain active—use your brain for calculation, remembering phone numbers, locating shops, friends, places. Remember the brain is an app! Do not depend on smartphones, otherwise the phone will remain smart and the brain becomes lazy!

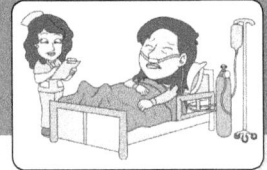
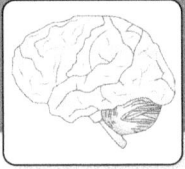

# CHAPTER 22

# Confusion and Coma

Consciousness includes awareness of self and environment.

The anatomical substrate for arousal is ascending reticular activating system and for awareness, cerebral cortex.

## ACUTE ENCEPHALOPATHY

### Confused Patient (and the Doctor!)

When dealing with a confused, disoriented patient, it is not uncommon to see the clinician equally confused! The symptoms of cerebral irritation are confusion, disorientation, delirium and is known as "acute confusional state", "acute encephalopathy" or "acute organic brain syndrome" (Table 22.1).

**Table 22.1: Acute encephalopathy—clinical features.**

- Reduced comprehension
- Attention deficit
- Hallucinations
- Memory
- Speech involvement

As the disease progresses the patient becomes quiet. The doctor thinks that the patient has improved. A restless confused patient who becomes quiet may be getting back to normalcy or may be deteriorating to an unconscious state! Be careful to assess the situation (Table 22.2).

**Table 22.2: Clinical features of cerebral depression.**

- Drowsiness
- Stupor
- Coma

Coma is a state of unarousable unconsciousness.

In senior citizens, the causes of encephalopathy are largely due to medical disorders (Table 22.3).

> **Table 22.3: Common causes of acute encephalopathy in senior citizens.**
> - Electrolyte disturbances (hyponatremia)
> - Metabolic disturbances (hypoglycemia, hypoxemia)
> - Drug induced (anticholinergics and sedatives)
> - Systemic infections like chest infection, urinary tract infection can also cause higher function disturbances without directly involving the nervous system

The direct cerebral involvement is encephalitis global/generalized, (e.g. viral encephalitis, pyogenic meningoencephalitis) or focal (e.g. herpes simplex encephalitis).

The causes mentioned in coma are applicable to acute encephalopathy and hence the *approach to diagnosis are on the same lines.*

***Case History of 65-year-old male:*** New onset seizures for which he was investigated but the particular cause could not be detected. A week later, he developed confusion and disorientation for which he was reinvestigated, for encephalopathy. The earlier seizure was thought to be due to the same disease. When examined he had symptoms of encephalopathy and the drug list showed that he was started on valproate 500 mg tds. The drug was stopped for 48 hours and reintroduced in a smaller dose of 200 mg bd; he improved dramatically.

***Diagnosis:*** Valproate encephalopathy.

***Message:*** Valproate encephalopathy occurs due to toxic doses and one should always start any antiepileptic drug in a small dose and build it up gradually if required.

## COMA

The anatomical substrate for unconscious state is "focal" lesion of the reticular formation in upper brainstem or lower diencephalon, or "global" involvement of bilateral cerebral hemispheres. By this implication unilateral cerebral involvement per se, as in stroke, does not cause altered consciousness. Patients with dense hemiplegia are often fully awake. The unconscious state in a stroke is either due to space occupying lesion with the midline shift or due to edema spreading through the corpus callosum to the other hemisphere.

One of the daunting tasks for the clinician is to analyze a case of coma which is an absolute medical emergency. Sticking to a few basic principles during the clinical approach will go a long way in helping the patient.

History of onset, duration, progress, fluctuating level of consciousness requires to be elicited. Acute onset is suggestive of stroke/head injury, while subacute progressive state has several causes. Comorbid condition—hypertension, diabetes, endocrine dysfunction, organ dysfunction (hepatic, renal) along *with drug list.* History of head injury, convulsions, drug poisoning, alcohol abuse to be looked into. A detailed history from the person who first observed the patient in unconscious state is very crucial.

**Examination of a Comatose Patient:** In general ICU (intensive care unit) many of the vital parameters (heart rate, blood pressure, pulse, ECG) are assessed by machines, and by repeated lab investigations (glucose, sodium, arterial blood gases, etc.). However, neurological evaluation is possible only by human interaction and the doctor should go to the patient's bedside to assess the neurological status!

Glasgow coma scale (GCS) was introduced for assessing the level of consciousness in patients with head injuries but is also being used in comatose patients with other causes. Unfortunately the GCS score is not representative of other causes of coma. When talking of assessment of level of consciousness, it is better to be *descriptive* than use terms like "semicoma", "drowsy", "altered state of consciousness" or "the numerical values of Glasgow coma scale".

### Neurological Evaluation

1. **Assess level of consciousness:** The best response is when the person is able to follow verbal commands like "open your eyes", "put out your tongue", etc. and also able to move all limbs against gravity.

   When there are no spontaneous movements and no response to verbal request, observe for movements elicitable to painful stimuli.

   *Painful stimuli* is applied to the supraorbital area or over the sternum. *Make sure that patient's attenders* are not present when applying painful stimuli, because they may feel that you are hurting the patient!

   Record the observation to painful stimuli in the following descriptive terms:
   a. With minimal stimulus, head as well as all four limbs move vigorously—is a mild unresponsive state.
   b. The above movements occur only by deep painful stimuli—slightly deeper altered sensorium.
   c. Response to pain by moving his hand to the area of painful stimuli—purposeful movement.
   d. Response to pain, where the movement does not reach the area of painful stimuli—non-purposive movement.
   e. No response to pain but the breathing becomes quicker—is usually the least response to be observed for deep painful stimuli.
   f. Decorticate rigidity—response to painful stimuli with bilateral flexion of elbow, wrist and supination of arm is indicative of upper midbrain lesion (where bilateral cerebral hemispheres are dysfunctional).
   g. Decerebrate rigidity—response to painful stimuli with bilateral extension of elbow, wrist with pronation is indicative of the lesion being in the lower midbrain.

2. **Ocular movements:** Examination of pupil and ocular movements is an important part of assessment of an unconscious patient. *The room should be dark and the torch should have a powerful beam of light!*

   When pupils are bilateral symmetrical and respond well to light, it is a good sign. When asymmetrical, in an unconscious patient, it may suggest intracranial space occupying lesion with early coning and brainstem dysfunction.

   Open the eyelids and observe for spontaneous ocular movements. Conjugate deviation of the eyes occur toward the hemispheric lesion, as in cerebral stroke and away from the lesion as in brainstem stroke.

   When spontaneous movements are absent, reflex eye movements can be elicited by "Dolls eye movement". Stand near the head of the patient and hold the head with both the hands, keeping the eyelids open; quickly turn the head to the right side and observe the eyes moving to the left; now move the head quickly to the left, the eyes should move slowly to the right. Similarly when the head is bent forward, the eyes move upward and when the head is bent backward the eyes move downward. These ocular movements indicate intact brainstem functions which means that the unconscious state is due to bicerebral involvement.

   When ocular movements are absent, usually the pupils too are nonreactive. However in drug toxicity coma, especially *phenobarbitone poisoning*, typically ocular movements are absent with brisk reactive pupils! which is an eminently treatable condition not to be missed.
3. **Weigh the limbs:** One can make a diagnosis of hemiplegia even in an unconscious patient by observing limb movement to deep painful stimuli. Paralyzed limbs do not move. By experience one can also weigh the upper limbs. Lift both upper limbs off the bed and feel the heaviness of the limbs (paralyzed limb is heavier); when let off, the paralyzed limb falls to the bed with a thud while the normal limb feels lighter and falls gradually.
4. Look for signs of **meningeal irritation** like neck stiffness, Kernig's sign. Note that these *signs may be absent* when the patient is deeply unconscious.

### How to Proceed?

At the end of examination one should be able to place the patient in one of the following categories (Tables 22.4 to 22.6).

If the systemic causes are ruled out, then neurological investigations—like MR brain, LP CSF analysis have to be resorted to and when electrical status is suspected continuous EEG monitoring should be done.

## Table 22.4: Unconsciousness without localizing, lateralizing features.

**Systemic causes**
- Systemic infection—pneumonitis, urinary tract infection, malaria, viral fever, etc.
- Metabolic disorders—hepatic, renal, cardiac, pulmonary dysfunction, hypoglycemia
- Electrolyte disturbances—sodium, potassium, calcium, magnesium
- Acidosis, alkalosis
- Drug induced—anticholinergics, anti-Parkinson drugs, sedatives, antiepileptic drugs
- Hypertensive encephalopathy
- Endocrine dysfunction (hyper or hypo)—thyroid, adrenal cortex, pituitary
- Recreational drug abuse
- Alcohol abuse

**Neurological causes**
- Encephalitis (viral)
- Electrical status epilepticus

## Table 22.5: Unconsciousness with lateralizing, localizing features, e.g. hemiparesis, cranial nerve dysfunction, asymmetric pupil, papilledema.

- Space occupying lesions—tumor, abscess, hemorrhage
- Parenchymal lesions—cerebral infarction, demyelinating disorders

## Table 22.6: Unconsciousness with signs of meningeal irritation.

- Acute meningitis—bacterial, viral
- Subarachnoid hemorrhage
- Chronic meningitis—bacterial, fungal, parasitic, neoplastic

Clinical examination in semi comatose condition may show asterixis—*flapping tremors* of extended hands—suggestive of metabolic or drug induced encephalopathy. *Multifocal myoclonic contractions* are suggestive of metabolic or anoxic encephalopathy following cardiac arrest.

### Investigations

If no evidence of a primary neurological cause, then investigate for systemic causes like urine analysis, hemogram, blood chemistry (sugar, urea creatinine), electrolytes, calcium, magnesium, metabolic profiles (hepatic, renal), serum ammonia, arterial blood gas analysis and blood culture when septicemia is suspected.

Toxicology screening for diazepam, barbiturates, anti-epileptic drug assay where suspected—T4, cortisol levels should be done.

In a majority of comatose patients the underlying cause is reversible general medical disorders which should be diligently looked into.

Once the systemic causes are ruled out, look for a primary neurological cause and investigate (imaging, CSF). When this too is normal, continuous EEG monitoring is required to detect electrical status. *Subtle signs like* eyelid flutter, facial twitching suggest electrical status epilepticus.

### How Safe is it to Perform an LP In an Unconscious Patient?

If the CT/MR scan shows space occupying lesion, then there is no question of performing an LP. When meningoencephalitis is suspected, if CT/MR is normal, then LP can be performed. If one suspects meningitis in an unconscious patient and imaging shows diffuse brain edema, it is preferable to stabilize the patient, with anti-brain edema measures and then perform an LP. The appropriate treatment should be started based on the clinical diagnosis pending the confirmation by LP. For example, if pyogenic meningitis is suspected start appropriate antibiotics. When one is not sure whether it is pyogenic or tubercular start both the treatments and after getting the LP reports, continue the appropriate drugs.

**Management of unconscious patient:** The immediate management consists of stabilizing the patient, with appropriate airway, maintenance of BP, oxygenation and ensuring an IV line for drawing blood for the investigations. The management directed to the specific diagnosis follows.

If a person is unconscious, for several minutes or hours followed by spontaneous and rapid resolution of symptoms following should be considered (Table 22.7).

**Table 22.7: Rapid regaining of consciousness—causes.**

- Epilepsy
- Head injury
- Hypoglycemia
- Poisoning, stroke (VBI)

### Fluctuating Level of Consciousness

When the level of consciousness fluctuates from being alert to drowsiness to alert state, it is usually due to systemic causes like metabolic, electrolyte disturbances. Fluctuating consciousness with minimal hemiparesis, which improves with the level of consciousness is suggestive of *subdural hematoma.*

Therefore, in practice, with fluctuating level of consciousness, if the CT head scan is normal one should diligently look for general medical causes (Table 22.8).

**Table 22.8: Fluctuating level of conscious—causes.**

- Systemic causes—metabolic, electrolyte disturbance
- Neurological causes—subdural hematoma

*Case History*: A 65-year-old male was admitted with left hemiparesis of 4/5 power with fluctuating level of consciousness. Past history revealed that he had left hemiparesis four months earlier. The treating physician concluded that this episode is only a recurrence of stroke. However in view of the fluctuating level of sensorium, CT head scan was repeated which showed a chronic subdural hematoma with a midline shift. The patient improved very well following surgical evacuation.

## UNCONSCIOUS STATE DUE TO "FUNCTIONAL" DISORDER!

*Case History*: A 35-year-old male IT professional complained of giddiness and fell down unconscious at work. There was no history of seizures and he was shifted to the emergency room of a nearby hospital. His blood pressure was normal and he was unresponsive. Routine blood chemistry, electrolytes, LFT, MR brain, carotid Doppler, ECG and echocardiogram were all normal. On examination he was unresponsive with no neurological deficits or neck stiffness. On trying to open his eyes there was resistance which showed that the patient was conscious! Detailed history revealed that his superiors had told him that his professional performance was not satisfactory. On hearing this he fell to the ground. While being transferred to the hospital he kept mumbling to himself. The clinical diagnosis is "functional" and all the investigations done were unnecessary and expensive! It is important to clinically diagnose the condition before ordering for a long list of investigations!

The following clinical states to be identified, which have different causes and prognosis (Tables 22.9 to 22.11).

### Table 22.9: Brainstem dysfunction—clinical features.
- Unconscious patient with no response to deep painful stimuli
- Frozen eyeballs, dilated non-reactive pupil
- Absent corneal reflex
- Absent gag reflex
- No spontaneous breathing (patient on ventilator)

Brain death to be considered, *if irreversibility of the condition* is diagnosed. Identification of brain death has assumed importance because of organ donation which can save several lives.

### Table 22.10: Persistent vegetative state (PVS).
- No signs of awareness, self or surroundings
- Opens eyes, rolls eyes, grunts, groans
- Automatism—groaning, grunting, swallowing
- Causes—diffuse cerebral dysfunction, e.g. head injury

Cardiac arrest—revival, terminal Alzheimer's disease

### Table 22.11: Locked in syndrome (awake brain locked in immobile body).

- Patient is fully conscious, aware of self and surroundings
- Cannot speak, cannot move limbs, cannot grunt and groan
- Communication only by blinking of eye and vertical eye movements

**Causes:**
- Ventral pons lesion, e.g. pontine infarction, myelinolysis
- GBS, periodic paralysis

# CHAPTER 23

# Meningoencephalitis

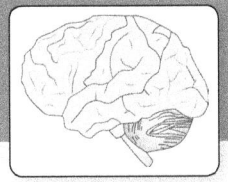

Meninges are the most pain sensitive structures and hence *severe headache* is the primary symptom of meningitis.

When the underlying brain is involved, symptoms of "encephalopathy" appear—disorientation, altered sensorium and seizures. Even though in both situations meninges and encephalon are involved (meningoencephalitis) the term meningitis or encephalitis are used depending on which symptoms predominate (Table 23.1).

**Table 23.1: Differentiating features of meningitis and encephalitis.**

| | *Meningitis* | *Encephalitis* |
|---|---|---|
| Clinical features | ❏ Fever<br>❏ Conscious<br>❏ Severe headache<br>❏ Vomiting<br>❏ Neck stiffness | ❏ Fever<br>❏ Altered sensorium<br>❏ Seizures<br>❏ Hemiparesis |
| Common causes | Pyogenic—meningococcus, pneumococcus, H. influenza<br>Chronic—TBM, fungal, carcinomatous | ❏ Viral encephalitis |
| CSF | Diagnostic abnormalities (Table 23.2) | Normal/nonspecific abnormalities |

**Meningitis:** The diagnosis of meningitis is arrived at if there is a combination of fever, headache, vomiting and neck stiffness. Acute meningitis can be due to bacterial (pneumococcal, meningococcal) or viral infections. If it is subacute or chronic the commonest cause is tuberculosis followed by fungal and carcinomatous meningitis.

**Encephalitis:** Here, there is direct brain involvement, clinically manifesting with behavioral abnormalities, altered sensorium and seizures.

## CSF Examination

The gold standard for the diagnosis of meningitis is cerebrospinal fluid (CSF) examination. It is very difficult to convince the patient and relatives for a lumbar puncture (LP) though they are more easily convinced for coronary stenting! The CSF should be collected in three bottles of 5 ml each where the

1st bottle is used for routine analysis, the 2nd one for PCR, antigen, antibody, etc. and the 3rd sample for further evaluation when needed. 2 or 3 ml of CSF is very inadequate!

The examination of CSF starts from appearance, which most often is not mentioned in the report! The interpretation is valued only if the CSF is clear. If it is blood tinged then the reports of cell count will be distorted. The tubercular/cysticercus antibodies which will normally be found in the blood may find their way into the traumatic CSF giving rise to wrong interpretation. Therefore, it is mandatory to start the report with the appearance of CSF.

Traumatic CSF should be differentiated from genuine hemorrhagic CSF, seen in primary subarachnoid hemorrhage. Presence of several antibodies in CSF (e.g. TB, oligoclonal bands) in traumatic hemorrhage has no clinical significance, as it only reflects the serum values (Table 23.2).

**Table 23.2: Differentiation of traumatic from subarachnoid hemorrhage.**

| | Traumatic CSF | Primary subarachnoid hemorrhage |
|---|---|---|
| Appearance | Hazy, pink | Red |
| Appearance in the 3rd bottle of CSF | Clearer | Uniformly blood stained |
| Presence of blood clot | + | - |
| Centrifuge CSF | Clear upper part as RBC settles down | Supernatant xanthochromia +/- (naked eye/spectro-photometry) |
| CT head scan | Normal | Subarachnoid hemorrhage |

Further analysis consists of protein, sugar and cell count (Table 23.3). It is prudent, particularly in diabetic patients, to draw blood for estimation of glucose just before doing a lumbar puncture. This is because if blood is drawn after the LP the blood glucose may go up because of the stress and anxiety of lumbar puncture. If the blood glucose is 200 and CSF glucose is 50 it is low sugar and pathological; however, if the blood sugar is not estimated and only the CSF sugar is 50 mg it is within normal limits! The cell count and the morphology of the cell must be looked into at the earliest—within two hours of drawing the CSF. If the CSF is drawn in the evening and the count is done next morning it will be very low as the cells would have degenerated thus giving a wrong report. Today there are many tests which can be done on CSF like TB PCR, TB antibody, Herpes simplex virus PCR and antibody, oligoclonal bands for multiple sclerosis. There are several other tests to detect various viruses which may not be of practical relevance when there is no specific treatment. There is a list of tests—Meningoencephalitis panel —which include bacterial, fungal and viral causes.

### Table 23.3: CSF finding in meningitis.

| Disease | Appearance | Protein mg/100 ml | Glucose mg/100 ml | Cell count/ cumm | Any other |
|---|---|---|---|---|---|
| Normal | Clear | 20–40 | 40–60 | 0–5 L | Nil |
| Pyogenic meningitis | Cloudy | 150–300 | <20 | 100–1000 P | Gram stain, and culture to identify bacteria |
| TB meningitis | Clear or hazy | 100–1000 | <30 | 100–400 L | AFB stain TB PCR, TB culture |
| Fungal meningitis | Clear | 100–200 | <40 | 50–200 L | India ink stain Fungal culture |
| Viral meningitis | Clear | 60–100 | Normal | <100 L | Nil |
| Carcinomatous meningitis | Clear | 60–100 | Normal or slightly reduced | <50 L | Cytospin to look for malignant cells |

L: Lymphocytes.

## Acute Meningitis

***Case History:*** A 45-year-old male was admitted with rapidly progressive restlessness leading to unconscious state within one hour. On examination he was mildly febrile with gross neck stiffness and CSF examination confirmed the presence of acute pyogenic meningitis. With appropriate antibiotics he rapidly regained consciousness in the next 24 hours. Further history revealed that he had a similar episode of pyogenic meningitis a few years back. On enquiry it was found that he used to have intermittent watery discharge from the right nostril suggestive of CSF rhinorrhea. He now required investigation for cause of recurrent pyogenic meningitis. An MR scan of the base of the brain and additional CT of the base of skull revealed skull base defect. He was referred for surgery for correction of the defect.

**Diagnosis:** Acute pyogenic meningitis.

**Message:** Second episode of pyogenic meningitis should be investigated for a cause and treated appropriately to prevent another such episode.

***Case History:*** A 23-year-old male developed febrile illness with body ache and headache of two days duration which was treated as systemic viral fever. Headache worsened with added vomiting; examination revealed mild neck stiffness. Clinical diagnosis was acute viral meningitis in view of low grade temperature as against high grade temperature in pyogenic meningitis. CSF showed inflammatory response with 30 lymphocytes, marginally increased protein with normal sugar suggestive of viral etiology.

**Diagnosis–Acute viral meningitis.**

At times it is difficult to differentiate viral meningitis and acute manifestation of tuberculous meningitis particularly in children. This is because the proteins and the cell count are marginally increased in both, but usually the glucose is normal in viral infection and reduced in TB meningitis. When in doubt start antituberculous therapy *without steroids* and repeat lumbar puncture after 8-10 days. If the CSF returns to normal, it is viral infection, as TBM, in spite of specific therapy, does not normalize the CSF values until 4-6 weeks of treatment.

## Chronic Meningitis

***Case History:*** A 28-year-old female presented with constant, progressively worsening global headache spreading over to the neck, of one month duration, with recent vomiting whenever the headache increased. CT head scan and MR brain including MR venogram were normal. The patient was being treated for chronic tension/migraine headache. Neurological examination was normal, and there was no neck stiffness. In view of *progressive worsening of headache with vomiting* and a normal brain imaging one should consider chronic meningitis. The CSF analysis showed clear CSF, increased protein, decreased sugar and 80-100 lymphocytes per cumm.

**Diagnosis—TB meningitis.**

***Message:*** Chronic headache, when progressive, should be investigated for chronic meningitis when imaging of the brain is normal. There is reluctance on the part of patient and doctor for LP!

Imaging in TB meningitis may show enhancement of meninges basal exudates, hydrocephalus depending on the stage of illness (Fig. 23.1). However the final diagnosis is by CSF examination.

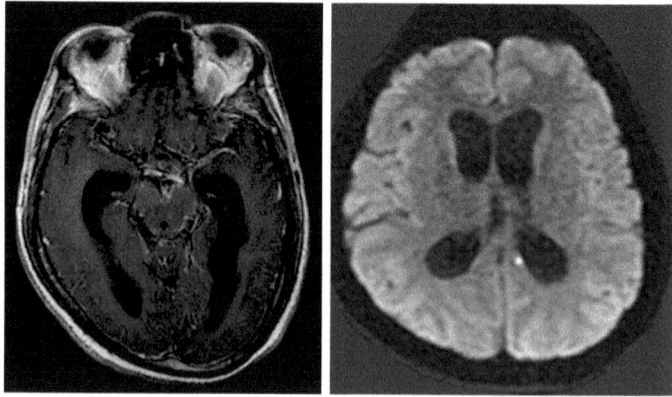

Fig. 23.1: MR brain—TB meningitis with hydrocephalus.

## Common Causes of Chronic Meningitis

In India, chronic meningitis is treated as *TBM* until an alternate cause is detected. It is very difficult to isolate TB bacilli in CSF because of the small number of bacteria. However, TB PCR if positive may help the diagnosis. It should be remembered that mere presence of TB PCR in CSF without a clinical diagnosis of chronic meningitis is non-contributory.

The other causes of chronic meningitis are: (i) *cryptococcal meningitis* (easily diagnosed by India ink staining of CSF smear, anaerobic culture of CSF) more common in immuneocompromised state like HIV infection; (ii) *Carcinomatous meningitis*. Here you have to chase the diagnosis, by *repeated LP and drawing a large volume of CSF* (20-30 ml) for cytospin and the slide must be examined by a person who can detect malignant cells in CSF, i.e. cytologist.

**Case History:** A 65-year-old male presented with chronic progressive headache of 3 months duration; no vomiting, no fever, clinical exam normal, brain imaging normal, no comorbid illness. LP CSF showed slight rise in protein with normal sugar and 20-30 lymphocytes, was started on antituberculous therapy, with no relief of headache. In subsequent two LPs, obtaining larger volumes of CSF with cytospin, malignant cells were detected—probably bronchogenic carcinoma with secondary spread to meninges.

*Diagnosis*: **Carcinomatous meningitis.**

*Message*: When chronic meningitis does not respond to antituberculous therapy one should diligently search for other causes—fungal, carcinomatous.

## ENCEPHALITIS

The clinical features are headache, seizures, altered sensorium with a background of febrile illness. There are no lateralizing, localizing neurologic signs and neck rigidity is absent. Once the systemic causes are ruled out, imaging of brain (CT/MR) followed by CSF examination should be done.

Encephalopathy due to systemic disorders are much more common and eminently treatable. The distinguishing feature is normal CSF in encephalopathy and inflammatory response in encephalitis (Table 23.4). Presence of fever may be a clinical pointer for encephalitis, but systemic febrile illness also causes encephalopathy. When confused, repeat CSF examination.

**Table 23.4: Differentiation between encephalopathy and encephalitis.**

| | Encephalopathy | Encephalitis |
|---|---|---|
| Confusion<br>Disorientation<br>Altered sensorium | + | + |
| Fever | -/+ | + |
| Generalised seizure | + | + |
| Partial (focal) seizure | - | + |
| Metabolic derangement | + | - |
| Neck stiffness | - | +/- |
| Neurodeficit (hemiparesis) | - | +/- |
| EEG abnormality | Generalized | Focal/generalized |
| MR brain | Normal | Normal/abnormal |
| CSF | Normal | Abnormal |
| Causes | Metabolic, toxic, electrolyte disturbance | Infective (pyogenic, viral, tuberculous) |

### Generalised Encephalitis

***Case History:*** A 20-year-old male reported with fever, body pain, headache, vomiting, generalized seizures and altered sensorium. There were no focal neurological signs and no signs of meningeal irritation.

Clinical diagnosis—encephalitis, in view of febrile onset, probably viral in view of systemic symptoms of body pain, myalgia. CSF showed slight rise in protein and lymphocytosis with normal sugar.

This is a picture of acute viral encephalitis seen commonly due to Japanese encephalitis virus, dengue fever.

***Diagnosis:*** Viral encephalitis.

### Focal Encephalitis

***Case History:*** A 30-year-old male was admitted in a *conscious state* with history of confusion, disorientation, incoherent talking and partial seizures of 3 days duration with a background of a febrile illness. A diagnosis of encephalitis (in view of fever, encephalitis symptoms) was made and patient was being investigated. The important point here is to distinguish generalized encephalitis from focal encephalitis (Table 23.5). In generalized encephalitis (which can be due to several viruses including Japanese Encephalitis virus) the patient will have steady deterioration in sensorium—from confusion, drowsiness to coma. If the patient continues to be conscious but disoriented it is suggestive of focal encephalitis.

Here, Herpes simplex encephalitis has to be considered which is an eminently treatable disorder. The CSF remains non-specific with a moderate rise in cell count and protein; sugar is normal. The diagnosis is made by detecting Herpes simplex PCR/antigen in the first few days and rising titres of Herpes simplex antibody in the subsequent LPs. *The practical point is that one should not wait for confirmation of diagnosis, but start antiviral drug—acyclovir—the instant there is clinical suspicion.* Not infrequently, the CSF, Herpes simplex PCR/antigen, may be negative in the first 2 to 3 days of illness, which is a very crucial period for starting of antiviral therapy. Additional diagnostic help is from MR brain (focal temporal lesions) and

| Table 23.5: Differentiating features of global encephalitis and focal encephalitis. | | |
|---|---|---|
| **Clinical features** | **Global encephalitis** | **Focal encephalitis** |
| Orientation | Affected | Affected |
| Behavioral disturbances | Present/absent | Prominent |
| Consciousness | Drowsy—Coma | Preserved |
| Seizures | Generalized | Focal |
| Hemiparesis | Rare | Present |
| MR brain | Normal/generalized abnormality | Focal abnormalities |
| EEG abnormality | Generalized | Focal |
| Common causes | Metabolic encephalopathy<br>Viral encephalitis | Herpes simplex encephalitis<br>Tumors<br>Abscess |

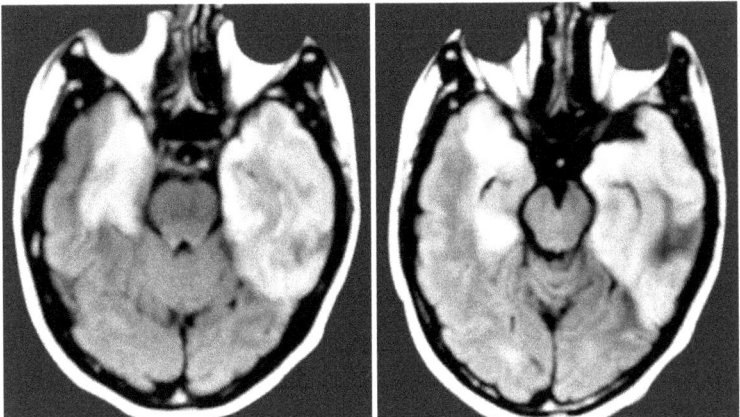

**Fig. 23.2:** MR brain—Herpes simplex encephalitis—bitemporal.

EEG (temporal slowing and seizure discharges). Repeat all investigations after three days and if results still negative withdraw antiviral therapy. If MR brain shows bitemporal involvement it is almost diagnostic of Herpes simplex encephalitis (Fig. 23.2).

### Autoimmune Encephalitis

This is a recently identified entity. *It is a treatable disorder* and hence one should not miss this diagnosis.

The ***clinical features*** consist of:

***Neurological symptoms***—Impaired cognition, altered sensorium leading to drowsiness and coma, seizures—partial or generalized (usually difficult to control seizures) involuntary movements like chorea.

***Psychiatric features***—behavioral disturbances, mood disorders, hallucinations.

The MRI and EEG are abnormal. CSF may show non-specific inflammatory changes, raised protein and cell count with normal sugar. The investigations include screening for systemic autoimmune disorders, neural specific antibodies in serum and CSF and screening for underlying malignancy and autoimmune encephalitis panel.

In clinical practice the evolution of symptoms over a period of several days, combination of difficult to control new onset seizures—usually partial—with cognitive, behavioral disturbances should be considered for autoimmune encephalitis if other causes are reasonably excluded. The treatment consists of iv methylprednisolone/plasmapheresis/IV IgG.

# 24
## Cerebrovascular Stroke

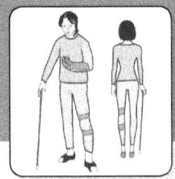

Stroke is a leading cause of disability and the third leading cause of death. One-third of the strokes occur in patients below the age of 65 years. Stroke, strikes suddenly, with focal neurological deficit like hemiplegia, as a result of a vascular event, an infarct or hemorrhage. Ischemic stroke constitutes 80–85 % of all strokes (Table 24.1).

### Table 24.1: Types of strokes.

a. Ischemic — Carotid territory
— Vertebrobasilar territory
b. Hemorrhagic — Thalamus, basal ganglia
frontal, parietal lobes
pons, cerebellum
c. Lacunar strokes
d. Cerebral venous thrombosis
e. Subarachnoid hemorrhage

### a. ISCHEMIC STROKE

The pathogenesis of ischemic stroke is a large vessel atherosclerotic disease common in carotid, internal carotid, middle cerebral, vertebral and basilar artery (Table 24.2).

### Table 24.2: Risk factors for stroke.

**Modifiable**
- Hypertension
- Diabetes
- Dyslipidemia
- Obesity
- Smoking
- Hyperhomocysteinemia
- Oral contraceptives
- Cardiogenic causes—atrial fibrillation, valvular heart disease, acute myocardial infarction

**Non-modifiable**
- Ageing
- Hereditary

**Stroke in young**—When it occurs in young patients, below 40 years, with no obvious risk factors, one has to investigate for procoagulant factors—Protein C, protein S deficiency, antithrombin III deficiency, factor V Leiden mutation, antiphospholipid antibodies, lupus anticoagulants, hyperhomocystinemia.

It is important to distinguish TIA/stroke of carotid system from VBI, as the carotid intervention is considered *only when* carotid insufficiency is the cause of cerebrovascular event (Table 24.3).

### Table 24.3: Clinical features.

**Carotid system**
Hemiplegia, hemianesthesia, hemisensory deficit, hemianopia, dysarthria, monocular blindness
**VBI (Vertebrobasilar system)**
Diplopia, dysarthria, dysphagia, ataxia, hemiparesis, cortical blindness

Ischemic stroke can be transient (TIA) which is often underplayed or enduring (completed stroke).
 i. Transient ischemic attack
 ii. Completed stroke

### i. Transient Ischemic Attack (TIA)

***Case History:*** A 65-year-old male hypertensive woke up in the morning and as he was going toward the bathroom fell down, was unable to speak and move his right upper limb. He was brought to the casualty within an hour. On reaching the hospital he was able to speak, could stand up with support and within a matter of ten minutes recovered completely. This is a typical presentation of TIA, *and is an emergency.* Patient's attenders, and doctors are quite happy about the recovery—*but it is an emergency—a forerunner for complete stroke.* This has to be emphasized and immediate admission and management is mandatory.

**Management** consists of assessing the risk factors (hypertension, diabetes, etc.), cardiac evaluation and appropriate treatment with introduction of antiplatelet drugs (aspirin, clopidogrel, and statin combination) to minimize recurrence risk.

This is to be followed by carotid Doppler studies and intervention if need be.

***Case History:*** A 52-year-old female had four episodes of sudden fall to the ground due to right lower limb weakness. Right upper limb distal weakness was simultaneously noticed. In another instance she could not open the gate and once the phone fell off from the right hand—all the episodes lasted for 1–2 minutes and occurred in a span of three months. On examination no neurological deficits were seen. Diagnostic steps are as follows:

*Step 1:* *Neurological deficit*—at the time of examination nil; but history suggestive of transient recurrent right hemiparesis.
*Step 2:* *Anatomical localization*—left cerebral hemisphere, motor area.

*Step 3:* **Pathological diagnosis**—in view of transient deficits, possibilities are vascular (TIA) or seizure disorder.

**Investigation** for anatomical localization—MR brain, showed left fronto parietal glioma, which was confirmed on operation.

The transient episodes were partial seizures, with negative phenomenon — loss of power instead of **tonic-clonic seizure.**

**Message:** *TIA should be differentiated from seizures (Table 24.4).*

Table 24.4: Differences between TIA and epilepsy.

| | TIA | Epilepsy |
|---|---|---|
| Age | Later age group | Any age |
| Symptoms | Negative (paralysis) | Positive (tonic-clonic movement) Occasional negative phenomena |
| Onset | Sudden and entire half of body | Sudden, spreads from one part to entire half of body |
| Sensorium | Conscious | Altered sensorium |
| Incontinence, tongue bite | Absent | May be present |
| Duration | Several minutes to hours | 1–3 minutes |
| Associated features | Hypertension, diabetes | — |

## WHAT IS NOT TIA?

**Case History:** A 65-year-old male hypertensive, presented with episodes of "giddiness" over a period of two weeks, underwent carotid Doppler study which showed 70% narrowing of right internal carotid artery. He was subjected to carotid stenting which was uncalled for. *Isolated giddiness is not a symptom of carotid ischemia.*

With reference to vertebral arteries, one artery may be thin or absent in nearly 30% of the population and therefore the report of narrowed vertebral artery does not imply that giddiness is due to vertebrobasilar insufficiency. Isolated giddiness is never due to vertebrobasilar insufficiency, nor is giddiness a symptom of cervical spondylosis, contrary to popular belief!

**Message:** *Any giddiness is not a cerebrovascular event.*

**Case History:** A 56-year-old male hypertensive, on medication, while alighting from a bus after a long journey fell to the ground due to giddiness. He got up immediately with no loss of consciousness or seizures. His cardiac and neurological workup including MR brain was normal. The carotid Doppler study showed 50% stenosis of right carotid artery and he was asked to undergo cerebral angiogram. Here the diagnosis is postural syncope, resulting from sudden change of posture from prolonged sitting in the bus to standing and walking. With the diagnosis of syncope, *carotid stenosis is not causative*. Hence, there is no need to do an angiogram. Unfortunately in clinical practice any transient cerebral event is referred for carotid Doppler study. If the result shows stenosis, the patient is referred directly to a vascular surgeon who dilates the stenosed vessel!

Always ask yourself as to why has the patient come to me and are his symptoms explainable by the imaging?

***Message:*** *Syncope is not TIA.*

***Case History:*** A 60-year-old female hypertensive/diabetic patient was admitted to the emergency ward with history of acute vertigo, vomiting and imbalance on walking. With a diagnosis of "brainstem ischemia" due to vertebrobasilar insufficiency, MR brain scan was ordered.

Detailed history revealed that as she was getting out of the bed in the morning she developed severe vertigo with vomiting and sweating. She laid back on the bed, 5 minutes later she was able to get up and go to the bathroom and while washing her face with her head bent, she again experienced another episode of vertigo and vomiting. Patient was examined while she experienced the vertigo while turning in the bed. Jerky horizontal nystagmus was seen. Both vertigo and nystagmus disappeared within a minute.

**Diagnosis:** Benign positional vertigo. This does not require MR scan or the prescription of aspirin!

***Message:*** *Do not confuse benign positional vertigo with VBI.*

### ii. Completed Stroke

Sudden onset of hemiplegia is a common presentation. However isolated language dysfunction is another way of presentation which is often confused for "psychiatric illness".

***Case History:*** A 60-year-old female presented with acute onset of not talking to anyone and being withdrawn, however she was able to attend to her personal needs. On the second day she developed difficulty to walk but did not communicate her problem. On the third day she was incontinent, unconcerned and refusing to take feeds. She was a known hypertensive. CT scan was normal and she was being treated for psychiatric problems. Examination showed sensory motor aphasia with right lower limb weakness. MR scan revealed left frontal infarct involving the perisylvian region.

***Message:*** Even if CT is normal it does not rule out organic causes. The clinical diagnosis should be organic brain syndrome of acute onset in an elderly hypertensive and one should look for vascular causes. Acute onset of so called "psychiatric illness" may be due to language dysfunction.

Stroke should be differentiated from conditions which mimic like stroke (Table 24.5).

## Cerebrovascular Stroke

**Table 24.5: Stroke mimics.**
- Hypoglycemia
- Hyperglycemia
- Seizure—postictal
- Subdural hematoma
- Hemiplegic migraine
- Space occupying lesion

*Case History*: A 60-year-old male was admitted with acute onset of left hemiparesis. CT showed non-enhancing hypodense area in right parietal region—an infarct. However, the hemiparesis continued to worsen slowly over the *next 2-3 months*.

The onset of stroke is always sudden. The deficit remaining stable/continues to improve/never progressively worsens over a period of several weeks as in this case. This should alert to the possibility of a tumor. A repeat CT scan showed increase in the hypodense area and subsequent investigations revealed a glioma.

*Message*: Progressive worsening of hemiplegia is not stroke—it should be reinvestigated.

Not infrequently hemiparesis is confused with cervical cord lesions (Table 24.6).

**Table 24.6: How to differentiate hemiparesis due to cerebral from cervical cause?**

| Symptoms | Cerebral | Cervical cord |
|---|---|---|
| Facial paresis | Present | Absent |
| Sensory impairment | Same side as hemiparesis | Opposite side of hemiparesis |
| Associated features | Seizures<br>Headache<br>Altered sensorium<br>Cranial nerve palsies | Neck pain<br>Cervical radicular pain |

There are certain clinical differences to distinguish cerebral infarction from hemorrhage (Table 24.7). However, the definite diagnosis is by imaging.

**Table 24.7: Differences between cerebral infarct and hemorrhage.**

| Clinical features | Infarct | Hemorrhage |
|---|---|---|
| Past history of TIA | +/- | - |
| History of high BP | +/- | ++ |
| Onset | During sleep | When awake |
| Headache | - | ++ |
| Vomiting | - | ++ |
| Seizures | +/- | +/- |
| Rapid evolution | +/- | + |
| Rapid recovery | +/- | - |

## Acute Stroke—CT or MR?

If the clinical diagnosis is definite stroke, then plain CT head is sufficient to distinguish infarct from hemorrhage, as the management differs between the two. If stroke is due to hemorrhage it will be seen in CT, if CT shows infarct fine, if CT is normal, it is infarct by default (Table 24.8). Remember that CT is cost effective, fast and easily available. However, if stroke is doubtful an MR is preferable.

| Table 24.8: Utility of CT head scan in a patient with stroke. |
|---|
| ❏ Differentiates stroke from stroke mimics (e.g. subdural hematoma, brain tumor)<br>❏ Differentiates ischemic stroke from hemorrhagic<br>❏ If hemorrhagic—arterial from venous<br>❏ Location of the stroke supra/infratentorial, right or left<br>❏ Extent of the infarct/intracerebral bleed<br>❏ Secondary effects like midline shift, hydrocephalus |

## MR BRAIN IN STROKE

MR brain is not a single investigation but has many added imaging techniques—diffusion weighted, and an ADC is necessary to diagnose an acute and subacute infarct (Fig. 24.1). MR angiography may show occlusion of middle cerebral artery (MCA) (Fig. 24.2) or ICA stenosis (Fig. 24.3). Brainstem infarcts are better visualized in MR brain (Fig. 24.4) than in CT. A routine MR brain may not identify old bleed and hence a T2 star imaging will help identify this. In summary, CT plain is the choice of investigation as an emergency. MR brain with DWI, ADC and MR angio should be asked for more detailed studies when warranted.

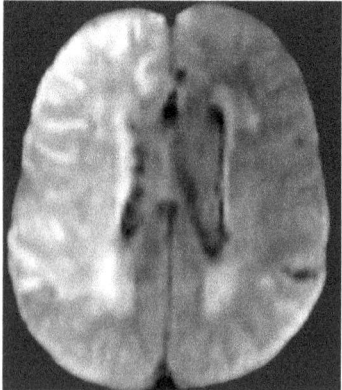
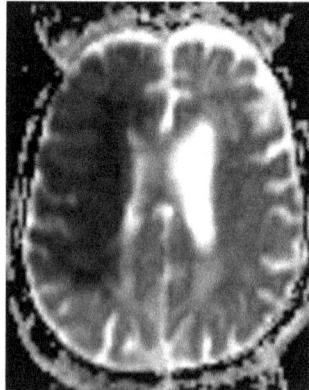

**Fig. 24.1:** MR brain—DWI and ADC right acute cerebral infarct.

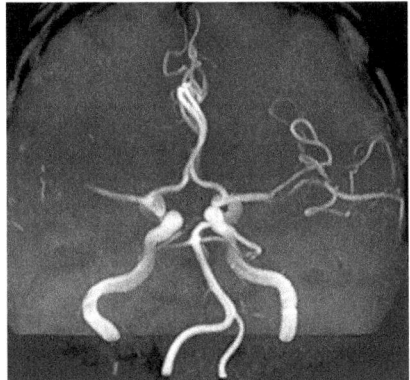
Fig. 24.2: MR angiography—right MCA occlusion.

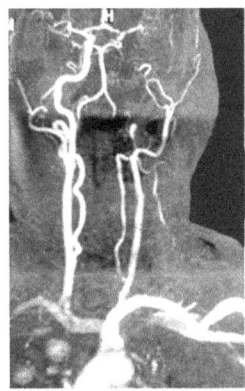
Fig. 24.3: MR angio left ICA stenosis.

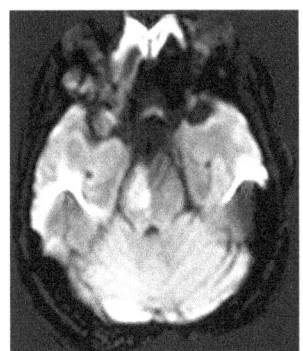
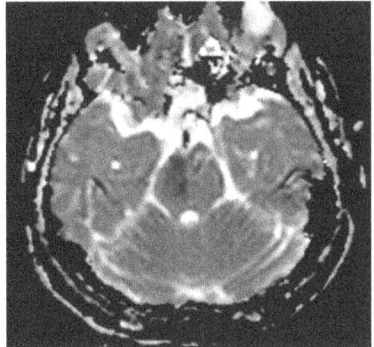
Fig. 24.4: MR brain—DWI and ADC acute brainstem infarct.

Cardiogenic stroke should be identified (Table 24.9) as the management differs—anticoagulants, not antiplatelets.

### Table 24.9: Cardiac causes for ischemic stroke.

- Non-valvular atrial fibrillation
- Valvular heart disease
- Myocardial infarction
- Prosthetic valves

### Principles of Management of Acute Ischemic Stroke

Stroke is caused by the abrupt interruption of blood supply due to thrombus blocking the vessel. The ideal treatment is to lyse the thrombus by IV TPA administration within 4½–6 hours of onset of stroke. In TIA, the thrombus occludes the blood vessel resulting in abrupt onset of hemiparesis and when the thrombus gets fragmented and disappears into circulation there is total recovery. Thrombolysis is an attempt to imitate this!

In cerebral infarct there is a core area of necrosed tissue which cannot be salvaged. Surrounding this is the ischemic penumbra, which can be salvaged by restoring blood supply by thrombolysis. The reactive brain edema further compromises blood supply which can be minimized by using anti-brain edema measures (Table 24.10).

| Table 24.10: Management of acute ischemic stroke. |
|---|
| ❑ Opening up of the occluded vessel (thrombolysis)<br>❑ Keeping the tissues in the penumbral region alive so that when the circulation is restored, they can be fully functional (neuroprotective measures)<br>❑ Reducing cerebral edema and raised intracranial pressure with anti-brain edema measures and surgical decompression in selected cases<br>❑ General medical measures |

### a. Thrombolysis

Thrombolysis can be intravenous, intra-arterial and mechanical—by clot retrieval therapy.

Stroke should be viewed in the same emergency as a heart attack as there are now therapeutic options available to limit morbidity and mortality from ischemic stroke provided they are administered within the first 4½ –6 hours. *Of course the earlier the better*. Procedures done in the first hour have better recovery than those done in the fourth hour. Creating awareness among doctors and lay people is required to transform the passive acceptance of stroke to an active intervention. The new terminology for stroke is "brain attack"!

Whenever acute stroke is suspected, immediately refer the patient to a *hospital which has facility for thrombolysis*. Do not waste time referring to a diagnostic center for CT/MR.

**Time is Brain**

The concept "time is brain" needs to be emphasized to utilize the effective treatment of thrombolysis. Efforts are being made to popularise this message through the word FAST among the lay people (Table 24.11).

| Table 24.11: Recognize stroke by FAST. |
|---|
| ❑ F — Face — Ask the person to smile<br>❑ A — Arm — Ask the person to raise both arms<br>❑ S — Speech — Ask the person to say a simple sentence<br>❑ T — Time — if the patient is not able to do any of the above three actions, immediately take the patient to a hospital which has facilities for thrombolysis |

Thrombolysis is done by intravenous administration of TPA (tissue plasminogen activator), within 4½ hours of onset of stroke. Beyond this time ischemic brain damage is vulnerable to hemorrhagic transformation. If a person has slept at 11 p.m. and is found to have hemiparesis when he wakes up at 6 a.m. he is not eligible for TPA, as one is not sure at what time the stroke has occurred! Further advances in the management consist of intra-arterial thrombolysis and mechanical clot retrieval, which can be undertaken beyond the window period of 4½ hours, particularly in vertebro-basilar territory.

### b. Neuroprotective Agents

Though much touted, agents like citicoline, pentoxifylline, Edaravone, cerebrolysin *do not have any significant* clinical benefit.

### c. Anti-brain Edema Measures

After an acute insult to the brain, be it a head injury or an ischemic/hemorrhage stroke, the reactive edema reaches its peak by 48–72 hours and resolves by seventh or eighth day. Wherever edema is contributing to the neurological status either in the form of motor deficit or altered sensorium, it can be minimized by anti-edema measures. The most important agent is 100 ml of 20% mannitol which should be administered in 30 minutes flat every 6 or 8 hourly for a period of 8 days *from the onset of stroke*. There is no point in giving 100 ml mannitol over 3–4 hours! One should be careful to avoid complications like an incipient left ventricular failure or renal failure. Other agents like Furosemide and Glycerol are less effective.

*When Should Surgery be Performed in Stroke?*

When an infarct or hematoma behaves like a space occupying lesion causing midline shift in CT/MRI and threatening coning and brainstem compression, *to save the life* decompressive craniectomy can be done. It should be made very clear to patient's relatives (as the patient is unconscious at this stage) that surgery is to save life and not to restore paralysis. One may save the life but there may be permanent disability and chances of the patient becoming bedridden! Surgery is very useful in cerebellar infarcts, cerebellar hematoma, and in young patients with cerebral infarct/hematoma.

*What Happens if Patient is seen Beyond the Window Period?*

When a patient is seen beyond the window period, intra-arterial thrombolysis and mechanical retrieval are effective in certain situations.

Generally aspirin, clopidogrel and statin combination is prescribed for first three months, followed by aspirin alone for lifetime.

### d. General Management

General management executed meticulously improves outcome significantly. That is the difference between stroke ICU from general ICU.

**Blood Pressure:** The blood pressure increases soon after the stroke to help pump blood into the ischemic zones which have lost the cerebral autoregulation. So, it is better to leave the BP alone for about 72 hours, unless it is higher than 180/120 or there is another indication like left ventricular failure.

**Blood Glucose:** The next important thing is to maintain euglycemic levels, i.e. if the patient is diabetic, insulin therapy for euglycemic level is necessary. IV glucose solutions should be discouraged, instead iv saline should be used.

### Temperature

Rise in body temperature adversely affects cerebral metabolism and contributes damage to penumbra. Hence, hyperthermia should be treated with antipyretics.

### Other measures

If the patient is bedridden with dense hemiplegia or is unconscious, prophylaxis for deep vein thrombosis should be initiated with low molecular heparin.

Where possible, indwelling urinary catheter should be avoided.

As patients with stroke have some degree of dysphagia, make sure that the patient is able to swallow normally before removing Ryle's tube.

### Not recommended

- Routine use of nasal oxygen is not indicated.
- Antibiotics should be used only if infection is present and not as a prophylaxis.
- Antiepileptic drugs should be used *only when seizures* occur and not as a prophylaxis.

#### Carotid Intervention

MR cerebral angiography tells us about the patency of the intracranial blood vessels, MR neck angiography, the status of carotid vessels. Doppler is more reliable in estimation of carotid stenosis in the neck. However, it is to be noted that Doppler studies are operator dependent, that is, the person who is doing the Doppler study must have good experience in regular carotid studies and correlate his findings with the surgical findings. MR neck angio over-reads. The main disadvantage of Doppler is that it cannot access the vessels near the base of the skull, particularly in short necked individuals. CT angiography is very useful not only to delineate neck vessels, but also intracranial vessels.

Carotid stenosis can be addressed by medical intervention—stenting or surgical intervention—Carotid endarterectomy.

**Indications** for carotid intervention—symptomatic carotid stenosis of 70% or more, e.g. right hemiparesis with left internal carotid artery (ICA) stenosis. If the patient has left hemiparesis with left internal carotid artery stenosis then it is asymptomatic stenosis!

If the patient has totally recovered from stroke, with independent activities of daily living, carotid intervention should be considered (Table 24.12). Remember that carotid intervention is for prevention of the next stroke and not to improve the present stroke. Therefore, if the person is bedridden with the present stroke, there is no need for carotid intervention, and hence no need for carotid Doppler studies!

**Table 24.12: Indications for carotid intervention.**
- Carotid intervention is to prevent the next stroke; not for improving the present stroke
- Symptomatic carotid stenosis of 70% or more
- Recovered from previous stroke leading an independent life
- To be done within 2–10 weeks

### *When is Intervention Required?*

The maximum risk for recurrence of the stroke is within three months and the peak incidence is during the first two weeks. After three months the chances of recurrence of stroke is same as that with best medical management. Hence for TIA, intervention should be done within a week and for recovered stroke within three months, preferably in the first month.

### *Which one to do – Endarterectomy or Stenting?*

It is the same problem as CABG versus stenting. Endarterectomy is a more preferred and appropriate treatment than stenting though the latter is less invasive. Endarterectomy is done in the neck. Stenting is done where endarterectomy is not feasible, e.g. high internal carotid artery stenosis that is nearer the base of the skull and in post-radiotherapy stenosis.

### *What is the Best Medical Treatment to Prevent the Recurrence of Stroke?*

The risk factors of the stroke have to be meticulously addressed—hypertension, diabetes, dyslipidemia, smoking, obesity. One cannot help ageing and genetic risks!

The present recommendation is to use the combination of aspirin, clopidogrel and statin (even if lipid profile is normal) for a period of three months and then continue only aspirin life long.

It is believed that the combination of these three drugs has a better prevention rate.

### *What should be the Dose of Aspirin?*

The literature says that any dose from 75–325 mg/day is a good dose. With higher doses, the benefits are the same but side-effects are likely to increase! Conventionally, neurologists prescribe 150 mg of aspirin per day. Some patients mention that they cannot take aspirin because of "gastric problem".

I tell them that the dose of aspirin prescribed is just 150 mg whereas for headache and fever one takes 325 mg three times a day! The single dose of aspirin can be taken soon after dinner to prevent any such gastric problems. Only in those patients who have endoscopy-proved active gastric lesion, aspirin should be avoided *till the ulcer heals*. In that situation the second best drug clopidogrel 75 mg has to be administered. Either of these drugs have to be taken lifelong.

*What is to be Done When a Patient on Aspirin Develops Another Episode?*

First and foremost the risk factors need to be controlled to prevent another episode. In addition if aspirin has failed, then, a second drug, clopidogrel is added and both have to be taken lifelong. A third drug dipyridamole is used when both fail. Oral anticoagulants are indicated only in cardiogenic thromboembolism as in atrial fibrillation.

### b. INTRACEREBRAL HEMORRHAGE

Hypertension is the leading cause of intracerebral hemorrhage and the common locations are:

Supratentorial—thalamus, basal ganglia, lobar (frontal/parietal) (Fig. 24.5).
Infratentorial—cerebellum, pons.

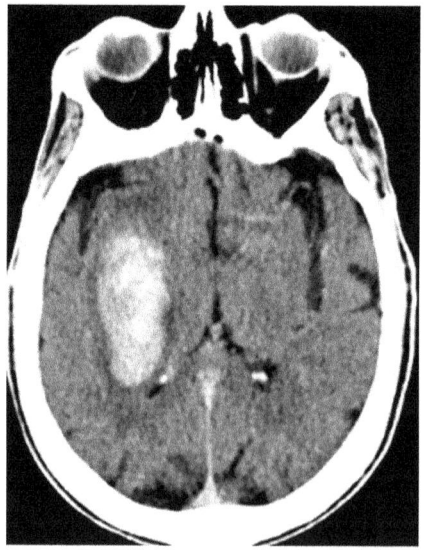

Fig. 24.5: CT head scan—right intracerebral hemorrhage.

Management is similar to ischemic stroke except that antiplatelet agents are not used.

## c. LACUNAR STROKES

Perforating blood vessels get occluded giving rise to specific neurological syndromes (Table 24.13) (Fig. 24.6).

**Table 24.13: Lacunar stroke—clinical features.**
- Pure motor hemiplegia—posterior limb of internal capsule, basis pontis
- Pure hemisensory deficit—thalamus
- Ataxic hemiparesis—pons, internal capsule
- Clumsy hand—dysarthria syndrome—pons, internal capsule

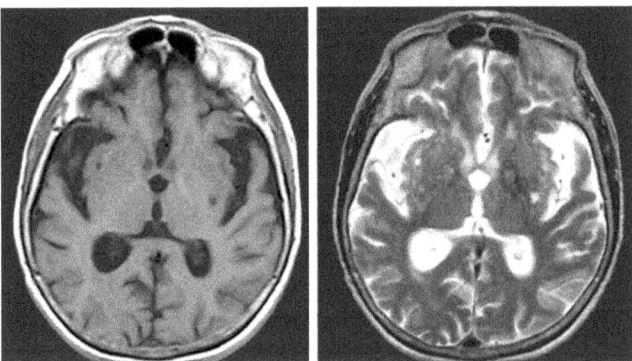

Fig. 24.6: MR brain—lacunar infarcts.

## d. CEREBRAL VENOUS THROMBOSIS (CVT)

There was a time when CVT was diagnosed only during postpartum period and confirmed at surgery/autopsy, occasionally by resorting to direct carotid puncture cerebral angiogram.

Now, with the availability of imaging—MR venogram—diagnosis of CVT is being recognized in both sexes and in different age groups (Fig. 24.7) (Table 24.14).

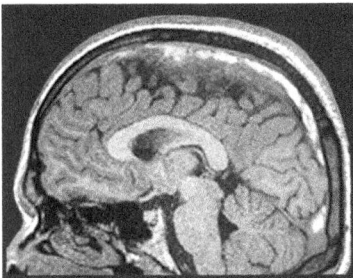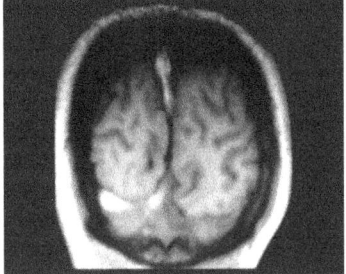

Fig. 24.7: MR venogram superior sagittal sinus and transverse sinus thrombosis.

**Table 24.14: Clinical features of cerebral venous thrombosis.**
- Progressive headache over a period of few days to weeks
- Seizures
- Blurring of vision, papilloedema
- Hemiparesis
- Altered sensorium

The routine sequences of MR brain may look normal, unless the effects of CVT on the brain are seen such as hemorrhagic infarcts on the surface of the brain. This should alert the doctor to ask for MR venogram which will confirm the diagnosis and the location of venous thrombosis.

In addition to the symptomatic management with antiepileptic drugs and antibrain edema measures (mannitol), the specific treatment consists of institution of anticoagulation like conventional heparin or low molecular heparin. The workup should include vasculitic workup and the procoagulant panel consisting of protein S, protein C, factor V leiden, antithrombin, antiphospholipid antibody, ANA profile and homocysteine.

### How Long Should the Anticoagulants be Continued?

At discharge the injectable medications are changed to oral tablets (warfarin or acitrom). If the procoagulant workup is negative, the treatment duration is for about six months and if it is positive, it is for an indefinite period/lifelong.

### Differentiation of CVT from Eclampsia

**Case History:** A 35-year-old female post delivery, on third day had headache which progressed over next four days, with visual blurring and partial seizures. She was normotensive during pregnancy, labor and immediate postpartum period. On examination was conscious with no neurological deficit. BP was 190/120, proteinuria + MR brain & MR venogram – normal.

***Diagnosis:*** Postpartum eclampsia.

It is important to differentiate CVT from postpartum eclampsia as the management is entirely different.

### e. PRIMARY SUBARACHNOID HEMORRHAGE

Abrupt onset of severe headache, vomiting, neck stiffness and altered sensorium are the clinical features of primary subarachnoid hemorrhage, usually due to rupture of an aneurysm.

Plain CT head scan shows subarachnoid bleed which gradually returns to normal by 2–3 weeks. To confirm, lumbar puncture should be done, 12 hour later to get hemorrhagic CSF. Once the diagnosis is confirmed, DSA (digital subtraction angiography) is performed to look for aneurysms and appropriately managed.

# CHAPTER 25

# Miscellaneous

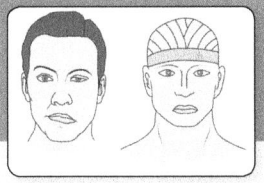

## BELL'S PALSY (VII CRANIAL NERVE PALSY)

Bell's palsy is fairly commonly seen in clinical practice and is often confused for a stroke if it happens in an elderly person.

The sudden onset of facial palsy is preceded by pain behind the ipsilateral ear. The paralysis manifests as difficulty to close the ipsilateral eye, difficulty to pronounce words, to rinse the mouth and to spit out the water from the mouth.

Examination shows paralysis of *entire half of face* including frontalis and severe degree of paralysis of orbicularis oculi (Table 25.1).

Management consists of oral prednisolone 60 mg per day for eight days (to be started within 72 hours of onset of palsy) and stop the medication abruptly. There is no need for antiviral drugs. Physiotherapy can be started for faster recovery. Protection of eye against dust, breeze and periodic eye drops are additional measures.

Table 25.1: Differentiation of UMN/LMN facial palsy.

| Symptoms | Bell's palsy (LMN) | Facial palsy (UMN) | Facial palsy—Hansen's disease |
|---|---|---|---|
| Distribution | Entire face | Frontalis spared | Patchy muscle weakness |
| Orbicularis oculi weakness | Significant, cannot close the eye leading to irritation and watering of eyes | Partial paresis, eyes fairly well covered | Significant palsy if the nerve twig to the specific muscle is affected |
| Associated features | Impairment of taste in anterior 1/3rd of tongue, hyperacusis | Weakness of upper limb, dysarthria | Sensory loss in the affected area for pin, temperature and cotton touch |

## RESTLESS LEGS SYNDROME

This is an eminently treatable condition that is often missed in clinical practice. The legs are meant for walking and they become restless when rested! A crawling sensation and disturbing pain in both the legs, particularly in the calf muscles, occurs when the patient lies down and is about to sleep. Characteristically, the symptoms disappear when the person gets out of the bed and starts walking.

The treatment is with clonazepam and antiparkinson's drugs like pramipexole and ropinirole.

## HEAD INJURY

Though head injury is a surgical problem, often patients approach a physician, hence a brief on the important aspects of head injury.

The brain is the content and the skull is the container, hence in any head injury one should assess whether the *content, i.e. the brain* is injured or not. (Table 25.2).

| Table 25.2: Head injury. | |
|---|---|
| **Types** | **Clinical features** |
| Head injury<br>❏ Direct brain injury | Unconscious, seizures<br>Hemiplegia from the *time of impact* |
| ❏ Indirect—Blood clot compressing brain<br>■ Arterial bleed (extradural haematoma) | ❏ Initially conscious—within 24–36 hours unconscious, hemiplegia |
| ■ Venous bleed (subdural hematoma) | ❏ Initially conscious<br>❏ Gradual (days/weeks) loss of consciousness, hemiplegia |

### Brain Injury

The clinical features which suggest brain injury are altered consciousness, seizure, hemiparesis. When these occur at the time of impact, then the brain parenchyma is *directly* affected due to injury.

However, if the patient was conscious at the time of injury and loses consciousness or develops hemiparesis after sometime it means "something" has happened between the time of impact and development of the neurological symptoms. That "something" is the accumulation of blood between the coverings (meninges) of the brain, secondarily compressing the brain — extradural/subdural hematoma.

### Extradural Hematoma

If the symptoms rapidly develop after a few hours of head trauma it has to be an arterial bleed, i.e. extradural hematoma which requires prompt surgical intervention (Fig. 25.1).

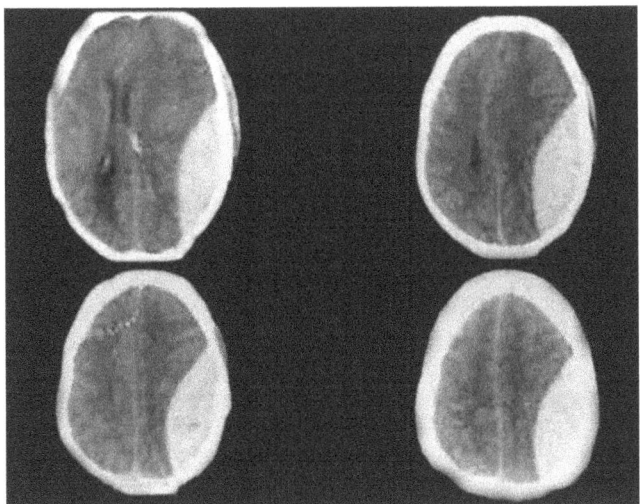

**Fig. 25.1:** Extradural hematoma.

### Subdural Hematoma

On the contrary if symptoms occur and progress very slowly say one week to 6 months after the head injury then it is a slow venous bleed, i.e. subdural hematoma (Fig. 25.2). This again requires surgical intervention but it is not an acute emergency as in the case of arterial bleed.

The practical implication is that after a head injury the patient has to be observed for 20–36 hours for any neurological deficit as this is the period when extradural hematoma may occur.

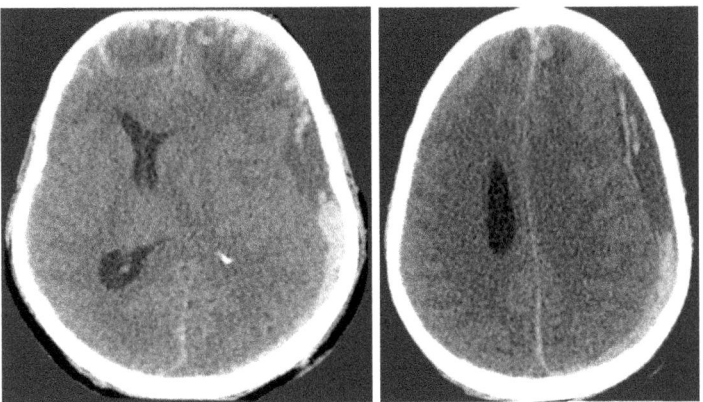

**Fig. 25.2:** Subdural hematoma.

***Message:*** The CT head scan done soon after head injury may be normal and needs to be repeated when there is altered sensorium which may then show hematoma; CT head scan plain is sufficient in head injuries as we are looking for blood clot and skull injuries which can be seen very well in plain CT scan.

Often patients are worried, saying that a lot of blood was lost from head (scalp) but was conscious and 20-25 stitches had to be put on the scalp! This is only a "container" (scalp) injury and not content (brain) injury!

***Post-traumatic syndrome*** consists of a host of symptoms like headache, giddiness, instability, lack of concentration, lack of sleep, memory impairment and others and is more common in trivial injuries where there is no loss of consciousness, seizures or other neurological problems. The CT head scan is normal is such cases. It is likely that the underlying symptoms of anxiety and depression come to the fore after the injury. Quite commonly patients complain of pain at the spot of injury whenever they are under stress. The management of such patients consists of reassurance and appropriate use of anxiolytics and antidepressants. Such patients may require psychiatric help.

## FURTHER RENDING

1. Harrison's Neurology in clinical medicine. Hauser S, Josephson S (eds), McGraw Hill, 2013.
2. HV Srinivas. Manual of Epilepsy—Medical Management and Social Aspect. Jaypee Brothers Medical Publishers (P) Ltd, New Delhi, 2016.
3. Neurology in clinical practice—principle of diagnosis and management. Bradley WG. Dariff RB, Fenichel GM, Jankovie J (eds), Butterworth-Heninann, Philadelphia, 2004.

# Abbreviations

1. AZ — Alzheimer's dementia
2. AAN — American Academy of Neurology
3. ACE — Angiotensin converting enzyme
4. Ach R — Acetylcholine receptor
5. AD — Alzheimer's disease
6. ADC — Apparent diffusion coefficient
7. ADEM — Acute disseminated encephalomyelitis
8. ADL — Activities of daily living
9. AED — Antiepileptic drug
10. AIDP — Acute immune mediated demyelinating polyneuropathy
11. AIIMS — All India Institute of Medical Sciences
12. ANA — Antinuclear antibody
13. AVM — Arteriovenous malformation
14. Bd — Twice a day
15. BP — Blood pressure
16. BPPV — Benign paroxysmal positional vertigo
17. C4-5 — Cervical 4th & 5th
18. C5-6 — Cervical 5th and 6th
19. C6-7 — Cervical 6th and 7th
20. C8 T1 — Cervical 8th and thoracic 1st
21. CT — Computerized tomography
22. CABG — Coronary artery bypass graft
23. CBD — Corticobasal degeneration
24. CBZ — Carbamazepine
25. CIDP — Chronic inflammatory demyelinating polyneuropathy
26. CISC — Clean intermittent self-catheterization
27. CK — Creatine kinase
28. CLZ — Clonazepam
29. CPS — Complex partial seizure
30. CSF — Cerebrospinal fluid
31. CVD — Cerebrovascular disease
32. CVT — Cerebral venous thrombosis
33. D1 — Dorsal 1st
34. D4 — Dorsal 4th
35. D6 — Dorsal 6th

| | | |
|---|---|---|
| 36. | DAT–SPECT | Dopamine transporter SPECT imaging |
| 37. | DLB | Dementia with Lewy bodies |
| 38. | DSA | Digital subtraction angiography |
| 39. | dsDNA | Double stranded DNA |
| 40. | DBS | Deep brain stimulation |
| 41. | DWI | Diffusion-weighted imaging |
| 42. | ECG | Electrocardiogram |
| 43. | EEG | Electroencephalography |
| 44. | EMG | Electromyography |
| 45. | ENG | Electronystagmography |
| 46. | ENMG | Electroneuromyography |
| 47. | ESM | Ethosuximide |
| 48. | ESR | Erythrocyte sedimentation rate |
| 49. | F | Female |
| 50. | FLAIR | Fluid attenuated inversion recovery |
| 51. | FTD | Fronto-temporal dementia |
| 52. | GB Syndrome | Guillain-Barre syndrome |
| 53. | GTCS | Generalized tonic clonic seizures |
| 54. | HIV | Human immune deficiency virus |
| 55. | HRT | Hormone replacement therapy |
| 56. | HSV | Herpes simplex virus |
| 57. | HTLV | Human T lymphocyte virus |
| 58. | ICU | Intensive care unit |
| 59. | IgG | Immune globulin |
| 60. | IV | Intravenous |
| 61. | JME | Juvenile myoclonic epilepsy |
| 62. | L4-5 | Lumbar 4th & 5th |
| 63. | L1 | 1st Lumbar |
| 64. | L5-S1 | 5th Lumbar and 1st Sacral |
| 65. | LP | Lumbar puncture |
| 66. | LBD | Lewy body dementia |
| 67. | Ldopa | Levodopa |
| 68. | LEV | Levetiracetam |
| 69. | LFT | Liver function test |
| 70. | LMN | Lower motor neuron |
| 71. | LTG | Lamotrigine |
| 72. | M | Male |
| 73. | MRI | Magnetic resonance imaging |

| | | |
|---|---|---|
| 74. | MS | Multiple sclerosis |
| 75. | MAO | Mono amino oxidase |
| 76. | MCI | Minimal cognitive impairment |
| 77. | MD | Doctor of medicine |
| 78. | MMN | Multifocal motor neuropathy |
| 79. | MMSE | Mini mental status examination |
| 80. | MND | Motor neuron disease |
| 81. | MSA | Multisystem atrophy |
| 82. | NCV | Nerve conduction velocity |
| 83. | NMDA | N-methyl – D - aspartate |
| 84. | NMO | Neuromyelitis optica |
| 85. | NPH | Normal pressure hydrocephalus |
| 86. | NSAID | Nonsteroidal anti-inflammatory drug |
| 87. | OPD | Outpatient department |
| 88. | OPLL | Ossified posterior longitudinal ligament |
| 89. | OTC | Over the counter |
| 90. | OXC | Oxcarbazepine |
| 91. | $PaO_2$ | Partial pressure of oxygen |
| 92. | $PaCO_2$ | Partial pressure of carbon dioxide |
| 93. | PB | Phenobarbitone |
| 94. | PCR | Polymerase chain reaction |
| 95. | PD | Parkinson's disease |
| 96. | PHT | Phenytoin |
| 97. | PSP | Progressive supranuclear palsy |
| 98. | REM | Rapid eye movement |
| 99. | SLIM | Society for less investigative medicine |
| 100. | TB | Tuberculosis |
| 101. | TBM | Tuberculous meningitis |
| 102. | Tds | Thrice daily |
| 103. | TIA | Transient ischemic attack |
| 104. | TPA | Tissue plasminogen activator |
| 105. | TTH | Tension type headache |
| 106. | UK | United Kingdom |
| 107. | UMN | Upper motor neuron |
| 108. | USA | United States of America |
| 109. | VBI | Vertebrobasilar insufficiency |
| 110. | VPA | Valproic acid (Valproate) |
| 111. | Yrs | Years |

# Index

Page numbers followed by *f* refer to figure, and *t* refer to table.

## A

Abscess 16, 25
Acetaminophen 57
Acidosis 159
Agoraphobia 47
Albuminocytological
　　dissociation 29
Alcohol 131
　　abuse 150
Alfuzosin 114
Alkalosis 159
Alpha blockers 114*t*
Alzheimer's dementia 15, 152
Alzheimer's disease 147, 152*t*, 154
Amitriptyline 36
Amphetamine 138
Amyloid neuropathy 135
Angioma 25
Ankle
　　dorsiflexors of 133
　　jerk 56, 57, 108, 133, 134
　　reflex 130
Antibrain edema measures 179
Anticholinergic 116
　　drugs 114*t*
Antiepileptic drug assay 28, 81
Antihypertensive drugs,
　　adjustment of 72
Antiparkinson's drugs 186
Antiplatelet drugs 172
Anxiety 87, 113, 138, 147
Aortic stenosis 70
Aphasia
　　global 84
　　types 84*t*
Arteries
　　temporal 31
　　vertebral 30
Arthropathy 49*t*, 56, 57, 57*t*
　　spondylotic 49
Aspirin 172, 182
　　dose of 181
Ataxia 41*t*, 45, 69, 87, 88, 172
　　psychogenic 92
　　vestibular 88, 92
Ataxic hemiparesis 183
Athetosis 25
Atonic seizure 94
Atrial fibrillation 171
Atrophy 130
　　cortical 30
Attack, acute 35, 37
Atypical parkinsonism 145, 145*t*
　　types of 145*t*
Auditory hallucination 152
Autoimmune disorders 131
Autonomic failure, primary 70
Axonopathy 27

## B

Back pain 55, 57*t*
　　postural 55
　　types of 55
Backache 25, 55

Baclofen 39
Bell's palsy 136, 185
Binocular diplopia 64
Biopsy, nerve 135*t*
Bladder
    dysfunction, symptoms of 112
    involvement 95
    neurogenic 112
    stone 113
Blindness
    cortical 172
    monocular 172
Blood
    glucose 180
    pressure 180
    vessels, narrowing of 30
Body pain, symptoms of 168
Brachial
    neuritis 53
    plexopathy 53, 132
Bradyarrhythmias 70
Brain 100
    injury 186
    MR 6, 22, 22*f*, 24, 25, 78, 78*f*,
        79*f*, 93, 99*f*, 151*f*, 153*f*, 166*f*,
        169*f*, 176, 176*f*, 177*f*, 183*f*
    tumors 150
Brainstem 89
    dysfunction 161*t*
    ischemia 45
Brandt-Daroff exercises 44*f*
Brisk reflexes 88
Broca's aphasia 84
Bulbar
    motor neuron disease 85
    myasthenia 110
Bulbocavernosus 108

## C

Calcium 159
Carbamazepine 39
Carotid
    Doppler 72
        studies 28, 28*t*
    endarterectomy 20
    intervention 28, 180, 181*f*

ischemia, symptom of 173
sinus hypersensitivity 70, 72
stenosis 72, 174, 180
system 28, 172
territory 171
Carpal tunnel syndrome 30, 132
Cauda equina 108, 108*t*
    syndrome 56, 58
Cavernous sinus thrombosis 68, 68*t*
Central retinal vein occlusion 61
Cerebellar
    ataxia 46, 87-89, 89*t*
    atrophy 89, 90*t*
    connections 89
    tumor 90*f*
Cerebellum 89
Cerebral
    artery, middle 176
    atrophy 153*f*
    depression 155*t*
    event 28
    hemorrhagic stroke 28
    infarct 175*t*
        right acute 176*f*
    venous thrombosis 171,
        183, 184*t*
Cerebrospinal fluid 29, 32, 163, 165*t*
Cervical
    canal stenosis 30
    spine, MR 23*f*, 98*f*, 100*f*,
        103*f*, 104*f*
    spondylosis 48, 48*t*, 51*f*, 52, 53
    spondylotic myelopathy 50*t*, 52*t*,
        53, 91, 101
Chorea 25
Circle of Willis 28
Clobazam 82
Clonazepam 139, 186
Clopidogrel 172
Clumsy hand 183
Coma 155, 156
Complex partial seizure 77*t*, 80
Confusion 155, 168
Consciousness 169
    assess level of 157
    loss of 94*t*

rapid regaining of 160*t*
transient loss of 27, 28, 69*t*
Conus medullaris 108
   lesion 108*t*
Conversion disorders mimicking
   paralysis 109
Cough 57, 70
   syncope 71
Cramps 111*t*, 130
Cranial nerve 12, 31, 66
   dysfunction 159*t*
   involvement 131
   palsy 64*t*, 185
   multiple 65
Credés method 114
Cushing's syndrome 150
Cyclosporine 138
Cysticercosis 25
Cystitis 113

## D

Daily living, activities of 8
Darifenacin 114
Deafness 43
Degenerative diseases 147, 152
Dementia 25, 146-150, 150*t*, 152
   frontotemporal 147, 152
   management of 153
   neurodegenerative 152*t*
   vascular 147, 151, 152*t*
Demyelinating disorder 29, 96
Dengue fever 168
Depression 147, 148, 149*t*
Detrusor hyperreflexia 116
Diabetes 131, 171, 172
Diabetic autonomic neuropathy 70
Digital subtraction angiography 184
Diplopia 69, 89, 172
Distal muscles 8
Dizziness 41, 46
   psychogenic 46
Dolls eye movement 158
Dorsiflexion, weakness of 56
Drop attacks 69, 94
   causes of 94*t*
Drug intoxication 150

Dural sinuses blood vessels 31
Dysarthria 45, 69, 83, 84, 84*t*, 89, 172
Dysesthesia 130
Dyskinesia 84
Dyslipidemia 171
Dysmetria 89
Dysphagia 45, 83, 84, 84*t*
Dystonia 84, 87
   focal 86

## E

Eclampsia 184
Electrical status epilepticus 159
Electroencephalogram 26
Electrolyte disturbances 159
Electromyography 27
Encephalitis 159, 163, 163*t*, 167, 168*t*
   autoimmune 170
   focal 168, 169*t*
   generalized 168
   global 169*f*
   viral 156, 168
Encephalopathy 163, 168*f*
   acute 155, 155*t*, 156*t*
   autoimmune 147
   hepatic 138
Endarterectomy 181
Endocrine dysfunction 150
Epilepsy 2, 27, 73, 74, 74*t*, 79*t*, 82, 94, 160, 173*t*
   classification of 76*t*
   diagnosis of 77
   types of 76
Episode, acute 100
Episodic weakness 111*t*
Extrinsic spinal cord
   compression 114
Eye movements 63
   testing of 63
Eyelids 158

## F

Facial palsy 185, 185*t*
Fasciculations 107, 130

Febrile seizure 75
Fever 168
 viral 159
Fluctuating motor weakness 88
Fluorosis 101
Folic acid deficiencies 147, 150
Foot drop 133*t*

## G

Gabapentin 39
Gait
 ataxia 46, 89*t*, 90, 91
 circumduction 87
 disorder 94
  types of 87*t*
 freezing 94
 imbalance 87
 spastic 87
 waddling 87
Genuine stress incontinence 116, 116*t*
Giant cell arteritis 40*t*
Glasgow coma scale 157
Granuloma, calcified 30

## H

Hansen's disease 135, 136, 185
Head injury 25, 160, 186, 186*t*
Headache 27, 29-31
 chronic daily 38
 classification of 34*t*
 cluster 2, 37, 37*t*, 38, 38*t*
 dull occipito-frontal 29
 localization 32*t*
 origin of 31
 progressive 25
 severe 32, 163
 tension type 25, 31, 34, 35*t*, 37, 37*t*
Heart disease, valvular 171
Heat intolerance 130
Hematoma
 extradural 186, 187, 187*f*
 subdural 16, 150, 160, 175, 187, 187*f*
Hemianopia 63
Hemiparesis 84, 159*t*, 168, 169, 172, 175*t*

Hemiplegia 63
Hemorrhage 175*t*
 intracerebral 182
 subarachnoid 29, 33*f*, 164, 164*t*, 171
Hereditary spastic paraplegia 101
Herpes simplex encephalitis 156, 168, 169*f*
HIV 150
Horn cell, anterior 87
Horner syndrome 66
Hot water epilepsy 77, 77*t*
Hydrocephalus 166*f*
Hyperalgesia 130, 134
Hypercalcemia 111
Hyperesthesia 130, 134
Hyperglycemia 175
Hyperhomocysteinemia 171
Hyperkalemia 111
Hypermagnesemia 111
Hyperparathyroidism 150
Hyperreflexia 116
Hyperreflexic bladder 112, 113, 114*t*
 hypertonic 112
Hypertension 171, 172
Hypertonia 88, 116
Hypoglycemia 69, 138, 159, 160, 175
Hypokalemia 111
Hypoparathyroidism 150
Hypophosphatemia 111
Hypoplastic vertebral artery 30
Hyporeflexia 89
Hyporeflexic bladder 112
 hypotonic 112, 114
Hypotension
 orthostatic 70, 72, 94, 130
 postural 72
Hypothyroidism 131, 147
Hypotonia 88, 89, 119

## I

Incontinence, types of 116*t*
Indomethacin responsive
 paroxysmal hemicrania 38
Infection, chronic 12
Intensive care unit 18

Internal carotid artery, left 180
Intra-abdominal pressure 116
Intracerebral hemorrhage,
  right 182*f*
Intracranial
  hypertension, benign 68
  pressure 25
Ischemic
  attack, transient 8, 72, 172
  optic neuropathy, anterior 61
  stroke, acute 177, 178*t*

## J

Japanese encephalitis virus 168
Joint position 130
Juvenile myoclonic epilepsy 20,
  25, 77*t*, 80

## K

Knee jerk 108

## L

Labyrinthitis, acute 45, 45*t*
Lacosamide 81
Lacunar
  infarcts 22, 30, 183*f*
  strokes 171, 183, 183*t*
Lamotrigine 81
Lathyrism 101
Legs, coordinated movements of 87
Lens 61
Levetiracetam 81
Levodopa 104
Lewy body dementia 147, 152
Limbs
  rhythmic involuntary
    movements of 137
  stiffness of 87, 105
Lithium 138
Low back pain
  acute 57, 58
  chronic 57, 58
Lower limb 124, 144
  intermittent claudication of 59*t*
  predominance 131

Lower motor neuron 15, 118
Lumbar
  canal stenosis 30, 58, 59*f*
  puncture 29*t*
  radiculopathy 56
  spine, MR 23*f*, 56*f*, 59*f*, 107*f*
  spondylosis 17, 56, 56*t*
Lumbosacral spine, MR 57
Lymphocytes 165

## M

Macular diseases 61
Magnesium 159
Malaria 159
Medial temporal sclerosis 22
Memory impairment 28, 146, 152
Ménière's disease 46, 46*t*
Meningeal irritation, signs of
  158, 159*t*
Meninges 48
Meningioma 30, 150*f*
Meningitis 16, 163, 163*t*, 165*t*
  acute 165
  carcinomatous 29, 167
  chronic 150, 166, 167
  cryptococcal 167
Meningoencephalitis 75, 163, 164
Mental status examination 148*t*
Metabolic disorders 159
Micturition 70, 71
Migraine 2, 25, 31, 35, 36*t*, 37, 37*t*
  basilar 36
  hemiplegic 175
Mini-mental state examination 148
Monocular
  diplopia, causes of 64*t*
  transient visual loss 61
  visual disturbances 61
    vascular causes of 61*t*
Mononeuropathy 131, 132
  multiplex 131
Monoparesis 25
Mood disorders 170
Motor
  deficit 57
  mixture of 123

neuron disease 15, 52, 52t, 101, 107
paralysis 102
system 12, 13, 119
    examination 13, 97
    weakness 53, 87, 88, 95, 95t, 107, 114
Movement disorders 25
Multifocal motor neuropathy 105, 105t
Multiple sclerosis, types of 99t
Multisystem atrophy 70, 72, 145
Muscle 84, 87
    biopsy 118, 119
    disease 27, 105, 118, 126t
    disorders 125
    neck 48
    occipitalis 31
    tension headache 31
    tone 105t, 115
    wasting of 95
    weakness 111t
Muscular dystrophy 15, 27
Myalgia 168
Myasthenia 27, 66, 84, 87, 88, 109, 110t, 111
    ocular 66
Myelitis 99
    transverse 96, 96f, 98t
Myelomalacia 30
Myelopathy 134t
    spondylotic 49, 52
Myocardial infarction, acute 171
Myoclonic jerk 94
Myogenic origin, proximal muscle weakness of 124t
Myogenic proximal muscle weakness 123, 124t
Myopathy 27, 66, 84, 87, 109
    clinical diagnosis of 27
    ocular 65
    statin induced 128t
Myotonia 87
Myotonic dystrophy 105

# N

Neck pain
    acute 51t
    causes of 48t
    chronic 51t
    management of 51t
Nerve
    conduction
        studies 30, 131, 134, 134t
        velocity 27, 27t
    palsy 64, 65
        lateral popliteal 133, 136
    vestibular 89
Neuralgia, trigeminal 39, 39t
Neurodegenerative dementia, types of 152t
Neurofibroma 30, 107f
Neurogenic
    bladder
        classification of 112t
        types of 115
    proximal muscle weakness 119
Neurological deficit 14, 16, 54, 97, 122
Neurology 1
Neuromuscular
    dysfunction 84
    junction 87
Neuromyelitis optica 100
Neuronitis, vestibular 45
Neuropathy 27, 131t
    demyelinating 27
    hereditary 135
    peripheral 30, 89, 91, 129t-131t, 134, 134t
    small fiber 130
    vasculitic 135
New onset sudden severe headache 32
Nicotine 138
Nocturnal enuresis 117
Nonepileptic attack 74t
    disorder 2, 73
Nutrition, consists of 12
Nystagmus 42
    central 43t
    gaze evoked 42
    multidirectional 89
    peripheral 43t

## O

Obesity 171
Ocular movements, examination of 12
Oculomotor nerve palsy 63
Oligoclonal bands 29
Ophthalmoplegia, painful 68*t*
Optic
 disks, blurring of 68*t*
 nerve 62, 100
 neuritis 62*f*, 62*t*
 neuropathy 62
  causes of 62*t*
Oral contraceptives 171
Orbital
 fissure syndrome, superior 68*t*
 pseudotumor 67
Orbits, MR 62*f*
Orthostatic tremors 139
Overflow incontinence 116
Oxcarbazepine 81
Oxybutynin 114

## P

Pain 53, 56, 57, 126*t*, 130
 burning 130
 neck 25, 48, 53*t*
 radiating 57
Papilledema 25, 68, 159*t*
Paralysis 95
Paraparesis 113
Paraplegia 95
 acute 96
 subacute 96
Parietal
 glioma, right 78*f*
 neurocysticercosis, left 79*f*
 tuberculoma, left 79*f*
Parkinson's disease 3, 20, 52, 53, 72, 87, 104, 105, 118, 140, 140*t*, 141, 141*t*, 142, 143*t*
 idiopathic 140, 144*t*
Parkinson's plus 145
Parkinson's tremors 139*t*
Paroxysmal
 hemicrania 38, 38*t*
 positional vertigo, benign 43

Pelvic floor
 exercises 116
 surgery 116
Peripheral nerve localization 133
Persistent vegetative state 161*t*
Phenytoin 39
 toxicity 90
Phobic disorder 47, 87
Plantar 108
 extensor 88
 reflex 133, 134
Plaques, demyelinating 22, 98*f*
Plexopathy 122, 131
Plexus peripheral nerves 87
Pneumonitis 159
Poisoning 160
Poliomyelitis 107
Polymyalgia rheumatica 128*t*
Polymyositis 27
 types of 127*t*
Post-traumatic syndrome 188
Postural orthostatic tachycardia syndrome 70
Postvoid residual urinary volume 113
Potassium 159
Pressure hydrocephalus, normal 93, 93*f*, 144*t*, 150, 151, 151*f*, 151*t*
Presyncope 41*t*, 46
Prophylactic therapy 36, 36*t*
Propranolol 36
Proptosis 67, 67*t*
Proximal muscle 88
 weakness 87, 119*t*, 124
Pseudodementia 148, 149
Ptosis 65, 66*t*
 bilateral 66
 unilateral 66
Pulmonary dysfunction 159
Pupillary reflex 68
Pure motor hemiplegia 183
Pyogenic meningoencephalitis 156

## Q

Quadriplegia 109

## R

Radiculopathy 49t, 51t, 56, 57, 57t
  diabetic 122
  spondylotic 49
Renal dysfunction 75, 150
Repetitive nerve stimulation test 27
Restless legs syndrome 185
Retina, detachment of 61
Retinal artery, central 61
Romberg's sign 46, 91
Roots
  multiple 56
  neurological involvement of 56

## S

Salbutamol 138
Sclerosis, multiple 16, 99
Seizures 69, 70, 70t, 73, 94
  late onset 25
  partial 25
  psychogenic 2, 73
  simple partial 80
Sensory 46, 57, 83, 84, 108, 119, 130
  ataxia 87, 88, 91, 91t, 130
  examination 14
  findings 133
  nerves 31
  neuropathy 89, 94
    symptomatic
      management of 135
  radiculopathy 89
  symptoms 129, 134
  tracts 133
Shoulder
  movements 53
  pain 53t
Sick sinus syndrome 71
Sigmoid sinuses 34f
Society for Less Investigative
  Medicine 3, 20
Sodium 159
Soft tissue abnormality 22
Solifenacin 114
Somatization, part of 55
Speech, normal 84
Spinal cord 16, 89, 100
  disorders 25
  infarction 96
  lesion 102t
  localization 133
Spinal injuries 96
Spine 48
  MR 23-25
Stiffness, neck 29, 168
Stiff-person syndrome 87, 105
Stress incontinence 116
Stroke 25, 160, 171, 171t, 172, 179
  acute 176
  cerebrovascular 171
  ischemic 28, 171, 177t
  types of 171t
Subarachnoid hemorrhage,
  primary 164, 184
Superior sagittal sinus 183f
Supranuclear
  gaze palsy 65
  palsy, progressive 145
  pathway disorders 63
Sweating 69, 89, 130
Symmetric distal neuropathy 131t
Symptomatic lumbar disc
  prolapse 25
Syncope 25, 69, 70, 70t, 72, 74t, 94
  cardiac 70
  cardiogenic 71
  neurocardiogenic 70
  situational 70, 71
  types of 70t
  vasovagal 70, 71
Syphilis 101, 150

## T

Tachyarrhythmias 70
Tadiculopathy 51t
Temporal meningioma, left 78f
Temporalis frontalis 31
Tendon reflexes 95, 107, 119, 130
  upper limb 53
Terazosin 114

Theophylline 138
Thoracic
　cord demyelination 91
　spine, MR 96f, 102f
Thoracolumbar cord 112
Thrombolysis 178
Thyrotoxicosis 138
Tinnitus 43
Tolosa-Hunt syndrome 68t
Tolterodine 114
Tonic-clonic seizure 80, 173
　generalized 76t
Topiramate 36, 81
Transcutaneous electrical nerve
　stimulation 58
Transient visual loss, bilateral 61
Transverse sinus thrombosis 183f
Tremor 25, 69, 137
　drug-induced 138t
　types of 137t
Trigeminal neuralgia, management
　of 39
Tropical spastic paraplegia 101
True vertigo 42, 43t
Tuberculoma 25
Tuberculous meningitis 29,
　166, 166f
Tumors 16, 25
　intramedullary 103f
　small benign 30

## U

Upper limb 124, 144
　predominance 131
Upper motor neuron 12, 118
Urge incontinence 112, 116, 116t
Urinary tract infection 159

## V

Vaginal delivery 116
Vague intermittent tingling 25

Valproate 36
Valproic acid 138
Vasculitis, diabetic 136
Venography, MR 34f
Vertebrobasilar system 172
Vertigo 41, 41t, 45, 91
　acute 45t
　common causes of 43
Vestibular
　gait disorder 91
　neuronitis, acute 45t
Viral meningitis, acute 166
Vision 60
　blurring of 25, 60
　double 60
　test 12
Visual
　and vestibular disorders 94
　field 68
　　defects 63
　hallucination 152
　impairment 60t
　symptoms 36
Vitamin
　B1 131
　B12 131, 150
　　deficiency 91
　B6 131
　D deficiency myopathy 125t
Vomiting 25, 45, 89, 91

## W

Wernicke's aphasia 84
White matter hyper intensities 30
Writer's cramp 86

## Z

Zonisamide 81

EU GSPR Authorised Reprsentative
Logos Europe, 9 rue Nicolas Poussin
1700, La Rochelle, France
Phone: +33 (0) 6 67 93 73 78
E-mail: contact@logoseurope.eu

www.ingramcontent.com/pod-product-compliance
Ingram Content Group UK Ltd.
Pitfield, Milton Keynes, MK11 3LW, UK
UKHW021831140426
5217IPUK00021B/1392